D1014819

The Magic of Herbs
in Daily Living

The Magic of Herbs in Daily Living

Richard Lucas

Parker Publishing Company
West Nyack New York

© 1972, *by*
PARKER PUBLISHING COMPANY, INC.

West Nyack, N.Y.

*All rights reserved. No part of this book
may be reproduced in any form or by
any means, without permission in writing from the publisher.*

Library of Congress Cataloging in Publication Data

Lucas, Richard Melvin, (date)
   The magic of herbs in daily living.

   Includes bibliographical references.
   1. Herbs. 2. Materia medica, Vegetable. I. Title.
[DNLM: 1. Herbs--Popular works. WB 960 L928m 1972]
RS164.L79   615'.321   72-6870
ISBN 0-13-544981-2

This book is a reference work, based on
research by the author. It includes his
studies as well as those of other authorities on various herbals. The directions
stated in this book are in no wise to be
considered as a prescription for any ailment of the reader. The prescription of
any medication should be made by a
duly licensed physician.

Printed in the United States of America

What This Book Can Do for You

In this book you have at your finger tips an excellent selection of herbal remedies which can easily be prepared right in your own home to give you the energy and go-power that will add sparkle and zest to your daily living. Many people in poor health have obtained astonishing results with the use of nature's medicines. Consider the following examples:

1. A woman suffering from painful bursitis of the shoulder decided to try a remedy obtained from the plant kingdom. She began to improve, and gradually movement came back to her shoulder. Before long she could raise her arm over her head. The simple remedy she used is described on page 227.

2. Mr. J.B., an insurance agent, had spent years at overwork, and business stresses had worn him out before his time. At 55 years of age he was ready for the scrapheap. His nerves were like those of a man holding a pneumatic drill and the twitching in his eye never stopped. Insurance was the only thing he knew, but in his condition he was totally unable to hold down his job under present-day pressures. Doctors advised rest, but months of that had reproduced little improvement. On page 109 you'll find out how an easy-to-prepare herb remedy put him back on the job with remarkable mental and physical stamina.

3. For over ten years, Mrs. M.L. endured frequent attacks of painful migraine headaches accompanied by dizzy spells, nausea, and vomiting. On page 171 you'll see how this woman became entirely free from migraine with the use of a simple herb remedy.

4. Mrs. E.M. reports that her eyesight was remarkably strengthened after eating the seeds which are described on page 00. Previously everything was a blur, but now she can read without her glasses. She adds: "Even my hair is getting life and luster back into it."

5. For three years a man had been under medical care for insomnia and nervous debility. Treatment with various drugs did not help. Induced to try nature's green medicine, he prepared a tea made from herbs; after one week's treatment he was sleeping well, and at the end of two months he was fully recovered. On page 163 you'll find a description of the herbal formula he used.

6. Mrs. D.B., 88 years of age, has a keen memory. No senility for her! On page 111 she perkily points out the herb that keeps her mind so youthful.

7. Seventeen patients with ulcer of the stomach or first part of the intestine were given the powdered pods of a certain plant as the only form of treatment. Fourteen of the 17 patients obtained immediate relief from their symptoms. Another of the patients had no relief for three days after starting the treatment, but on the fifth day his symptoms also disappeared. For the name of the plant that accounted for the beneficial results in these cases, see page 43.

8. A woman's husband had been troubled with constipation for years. A friend advised a natural remedy to be taken every morning and before retiring at night. This did the trick; he doesn't require laxative pills anymore. On page 75 you'll find the name of the remedy that was the answer to his problem.

9. For over five years a business man in his forties suffered from heartburn and nausea after meals, coupled with sharp pains in the stomach region, and a bloated feeling following even a fairly light meal. After all other forms of treatment had proved ineffectual he regained his health and strength with the natural program described on page 46.

Along with the extensive coverage of herbal remedies for coping with a wide variety of health problems, this book also presents a chapter on herbal slimming aids that can help you shed unwanted pounds without the use of gruelling starvation diets that make almost impossible demands on your will power.

In another chapter you'll read about longevity herbs and the ways in which they are used to help prevent the signs of aging and keep them at bay. Included are the health secrets of various people who have stretched their life span far beyond the proverbial threescore and ten to 100, 110, and over.

And if you are fighting a losing battle with the distressing problem of falling hair, dull lifeless hair or baldness, this book offers you hope as it contains a full chapter on selective herbs and natural foods to help promote a beautiful healthy head of hair.

Many marital difficulties are linked to poor sex relations. Starting on page 17 you'll find a chapter on herbs that can help tone up sex organs. Here you'll discover nature's golden nuggets of sex power; an ancient herbal love potion; an herb oil for sex health; a Chinese herb used for thousands of years as a sex rejuvenant; and a Mexican herbal aphrodisiac and tonic.

Another chapter provides you with a treasure trove of herb recipes for preparing your own beauty aids to help your skin look and feel years younger. This chapter covers cosmetics from nature's bounty—herbal facial beauty masks, herbal aids for specific skin problems, and herbal steam facials and cleansers. Ingredients are inexpensive, easy to prepare and use.

In addition there is a chapter on how herbs can be put to work around the modern household as stain removers, disinfectants, mold resisters, household cleansers, deodorizers, and insecticides.

Recently the subject of the supernatural has come into the limelight. Starting on page 133 you'll find a fascinating chapter which presents some completely new and startling information on the old legends and lore of plant magic.

Even in our modern age with its jet planes, space ships, satellites, and electronic brains, nature is still man's greatest laboratory and apothecary. All that is necessary to avail yourself of nature's herbal benefits is the know-how which you will find presented between the covers of this book.

Richard Lucas

Other books by the author:

Nature's Medicines: The Folklore, Romance, and Value of Herbal
  Remedies
Common and Uncommon Uses of Herbs for Healthful Living

Contents

The Magic of Herbs
in Daily Living

1

How to Use Herbs to Tone the Sex Organs

The use of love potions made from nature's own remedies is as old as mankind. Long before the emergence of the Hia dynasty under Yu the Great in 2197 B.C., Chinese healers were boiling the root of a plant known as *Jen Shen* and giving the brew to men whose sexual ambitions far outran their sexual capacities. In ancient Babylon women were munching candy made of sesame seed and honey for sexual health and fertility. For countless generations the Hungarian gypsies and the mountain-dwelling Bulgarians have been eating pumpkin seeds to preserve the prostate gland and thereby male potency. Centuries ago women were drinking beer made from honey and herbs to assure fertility and female sexual response.

For years the idea that these and other herbal folk remedies could deal effectively with a person's lovemaking problems has been regarded by medics as backwoods superstition and outright witchcraft. Recently, however, modern researchers have begun investigating, and their discoveries have led previously cynical scientists to re-examine their prejudices. And well they might. The age-old reputation of many plants for correcting sexual inadequacies can now be backed up by scientific proof.

The herbs covered in the pages of this chapter are not aphrodisiacs in the strict sense of the term, but sources of nutrients needed for building the health of the various sex glands and organs of the reproductive system.

SESAME SEEDS—GOLDEN NUGGETS OF SEX POWER

In Eastern folklore, the phrase "Open Sesame" was used as a magic charm for opening up a wonderland of riches. Perhaps the name *sesame* was chosen because the people realized that locked within this tiny seed lies a vast abundance of nutritional riches of exceptional value in human health. That they knew sesame was a remarkably wholesome food is apparent from their written records. One striking example, reported by the Greek historian Herodotus, credited sesame seeds with preventing the castration of 300 boys who were being forcibly sent to Ayattes to become eunuchs.

During the journey the guards stopped over at Samos, and the Samians, hearing of the fate in store for the boys, gave them sanctuary in the temple of Diana. The outraged Corinthian guards immediately cut off food supplies to the youths in order to force their surrender through hunger. But the Samians were not to be outwitted. They quickly originated a festival, which in part required participants of the choirs to stand around in the temple holding sesame seed cakes in their hands so that the young lads might grab them. The festival continued for such a long time that the Corinthian guards finally gave up in disgust and left the city.

Treasured Seed of the Ancients

Sesame seed was one of the most important spice herbs grown in the magnificent Hanging Gardens of Babylon. Throughout Babylonian history the seed was highly valued and its production a matter of royal attention. Seeds dispatched to important personages of neighboring lands were sent under escort of the most trustworthy guards. The seeds also became a subject of contract. One ancient tablet mentions a loan of silver and sesame seed; another records an allowance of food, drink, and sesame seed to be given to a man and his family.

The Babylonians loved the nut-like flavor of sesame and used the seeds in making cakes, candies, brandy, and wine. Women mixed the crushed seeds with honey and ate the delicacy to tone up their sex glands.

Sesame seed oil found favor in medicine, as a food, and in the preparation of perfume. According to Herodotus, it was the only oil the Babylonians would use. Because of its aromatic properties and its soothing effect on the skin it was highly acceptable for anointing the body.

Sex Power of Sesame Seed Candy Identified

Dr. Formica of Old Bridge, New Jersey, is reported to have successfully treated scores of married women for what he calls "housewife syndrome," a condition symptomized by fatigue, boredom with housework and bedroom "hanky-panky." Sometimes it is accompanied by nervousness, insomnia, headache, and backache.

The treatment prescribed by Dr. Formica is a drug, said to be the potassium and magnesium salts of aspartic acid. Now when we check into the food analysis of the candy made from sesame seed and honey which was eaten by the Babylonian women in ancient times, we find that honey is rich in aspartic acid, and sesame seed is an excellent source of potassium and magnesium. Blend them together and you have a rich supply of potassium and magnesium salts of aspartic acid—just what the doctor ordered!

Positive Sex Power

Dr. Formica reports that he obtained a positive result in 87% of his patients after four to six weeks of treatment with the prescription drug. He claims the change was astonishing. The women became cheerful, happy, alert, and sexually responsive to their mates. They also reported that sleep refreshed them as it had not done for some time. Grateful husbands called the good doctor and expressed appreciation for the physical and emotional improvement in their wives.

Dr. Formica explains that his treatment is not recommended for everyone, since chronic fatigue can be a symptom of disease or can have a psychological origin. "Housewife syndrome," on the other hand, is a condition in which there is no disease but a lack or shortage of certain nutrients which makes it difficult, if not impossible, for a person to function up to par. In these cases the prescription drug works admirably.

Make-It-Yourself Sex Candy

You can make your own candy of sesame seed and honey and thereby assure yourself of a rich supply of potassium and magnesium salts of aspartic acid. And in addition you get a bonus, for this delicious confection also contains ample amounts of vitamin E (called the fertility vitamin), along with other valuable nutrients—calcium, phosphorus, and unsaturated fatty acids (vitamin F) as well as associated lecithin so necessary for good health. But that's not all. Sesame seeds also contain 50% more protein than meat. Dr. Leathem of Rutgers University explains that the hormone (hypophyseal) produced by the pituitary gland is basically protein in nature and obviously needs this nutrient in the diet for its development. This hormone is a key factor to healthy activity of the sex glands.

Sesame Seed Candy

Place one cup of sesame seed meal in a bowl. Knead and work in small bits of honey. If additional flavoring is desired, you can add a dash of vanilla or maple, or you can work in small amounts of peanut butter. Shape into small mounds or balls, place on a cookie sheet and store in the refrigerator.

Here is another sesame treat to spark your vital power: Place two cups of sesame seed meal and ¼ cup sesame seed oil in a large bowl and stir until well mixed, then add two tablespoons of honey and a dash of vanilla. Continue stirring until the mixture is smooth, then add a few finely chopped dates. Shape into small pieces and store in the refrigerator.

Taste-Appeal with a Wide Variety of Uses

There are many other ways of fortifying your diet with these tiny power-packed seeds. For example, a thick cream called Tahini is made from liquified sesame seeds. This product can be obtained from your health food store. Nothing has been added, subtracted, or refined. It is a remarkable food, easily digested and in the bloodstream as energy in less than 30 minutes. Tahini is a good healthy substitute for ordinary cream or butter, which it is better to avoid. Mix it with honey and chopped nuts or dates and you have a delicious dessert as well as a quick source of energy. Or you can use it as a topping on potatoes, yogurt, vegetables, fruit, toast, salads, or as a sauce on fish or eggs.

Another very fine product is halvah, which is made of sesame seeds (including the oil) and honey. It has the consistency of fudge and can be obtained in various flavors: vanilla, chocolate, and marbled, or with chopped nut covering. There are some inferior grades of halvah on the market which contain large amounts of refined sugar or corn syrup, so be sure to read the label before making your purchase.

Sesame seeds alone can be used in a variety of ways. A small bowl of the freshly ground meal can be set right on the table, to be spooned onto foods as desired. The seeds are excellent in tossed salads and can be mixed with soups or almost any other kind of food. Dip slices of banana in yogurt and roll them in the seeds. Try sesame seeds instead of bread crumbs in casseroles. Sprinkle the seeds generously on cookies, muffins, rolls, puddings, fruit, and other desserts. The unique sesame flavor blends harmoniously and enhances whatever it is used with.

You can buy sesame seeds at health food stores, mail order health food companies, herb companies, and even at some supermarkets or corner grocery stores. You can obtain the ground sesame seed meal and halvah candy bars at health food stores.

PUMPKIN SEEDS FOR "HE-MAN" POWER

The use of pumpkin seeds for their beneficial effect on the prostate gland is as old as the ages. This favorite folk remedy of gypsies, Germans, and others, has now caught the attention of modern science. Dr. W. Devrient of Berlin, Germany, reports that he has been curing patients of prostate trouble by having them eat pumpkin seeds regularly. Here is a brief extract from an article he wrote on the value of this remarkable plant:

> There is a disease-preventive plant, little noticed until now, whose rejuvenating powers for men are extolled with praise by popular

medicine both in America and in Europe. Experience reveals that men in those countries where the seeds of this plant are copiously eaten throughout a lifetime remain amazingly free of prostatic hypertrophy (prostate trouble) and all its consequences.

The Importance of a Healthy Prostate Gland

The prostate gland manufactures prostatic fluid which nourishes the male spermatozoa and keeps them alive. If the prostate becomes enlarged it closes off the bladder, and pain, discomfort, difficulty with urination, and serious illness arise.

Certain Amino Acids in Foods Provide Relief for Enlarged Prostate

A new medication, not a drug but a nutrient which exists naturally in certain foods, has been successfully used for non-surgical treatment of the enlarged prostate gland. The treatment consists of a mixture of three amino acids—alanine, glycine, and glutamic acid. Doctors Julian Grant and Henry Feinblatt, who discovered the important medication, reported that patients with an enlarged prostate associated with urinary difficulties experienced prompt and dramatic relief after taking the amino mixture. They remained free of the symptoms as long as they kept taking the compound, but the symptoms would return if they discontinued the medication.

It may surprise you to know that pumpkin seeds contain the very same amino acids that are used in the professional medication!

Minerals That Benefit the Sex Glands

Chemical analyses of the healthy prostate gland and of spermatozoa (the male "living seed") show very high concentrations of zinc, whereas the amount of zinc found in the sick prostate is low. So it seems likely that this mineral is extremely important to the health of the reproductive system. Studies reported by Dr. Mayer show that in certain lands or regions where there is a widespread deficiency of zinc, the sex organs do not develop properly. Describing a group near Cairo, Egypt, Dr. Mayer wrote: "Their external genitals were remarkably small, with both atrophic testes and small penises; and they had no facial, pubic, or axillary hair. . . ."

Pumpkin seeds are just about the richest natural sources of zinc nutrition you will ever find.

The Magic of Magnesium

Magnesium is another important mineral found abundantly in pumpkin seeds.

Several French scientists have achieved remarkable results in the prevention and cure of prostatic disorders by administering magnesium compounds. One French physician made inquiries of those of his male medical friends who took magnesium chloride after they had read a report of its effectiveness in treating prostate trouble. He learned that four out of five of them had suffered difficulty in urinating, but after taking magnesium tablets their urinating disturbances had either greatly lessened or vanished completely.

Interesting data on 12 prostatic cases treated with magnesium was reported by another French physician, Dr. Chevassu. Ten of the 12 patients were completely cured and their general physical health also greatly improved.

In one of Dr. Chevassu's cases, the patient was suffering complete retention of urine and had been sent to the hospital to have his prostate gland surgically removed. However, Dr. Chevassu felt that in this particular case it would be too dangerous to operate, so the patient was given magnesium chloride tablets. Within a short time spontaneous urination occurred. The patient kept taking the magnesium tablets after he returned home from the hospital and has not had any further pain or difficulty with urination.

Dr. Favier of Paris stated that among the men who have been using magnesium chloride regularly for many years, none so far as he knows has suffered from prostate trouble.

Commenting on the use of magnesium compounds for the treatment of prostate disease, Mr. J. I. Rodale of *Prevention* magazine says:

> This is all right in an emergency, but in a program of preventing this disease, I recommend and have popularized the more inert form of

magnesium from the rock called dolomite. This is ground extremely fine and is available as tablets in all health food stores. Through my efforts hundreds of thousands are now taking dolomite tablets.

So in order to prevent prostate difficulties I suggest a program of pumpkin seeds and dolomite tablets. These can even be consumed by the very young as they do not pose any dangerous side-effects, but are helpful to the general health of the body.[1]

HONEY-BEER–A "HONEY" OF A LOVE POTION

The use of honey both as food and as medicine dates from antiquity. It is mentioned frequently in the Bible and in the ancient sacred texts of China, India, Egypt, and Persia.

In olden times the bride drank honey-beer for the 30 days directly following the marriage ceremony in order to assure fertility and to guard against female coldness. It is from this custom that the term "honeymoon" is derived.

The ancient love-elixir was originally made of fermented malt and honey, flavored with various aromatic and bitter herbs according to taste. Later the honey beverage was prepared with hops rather than malt.

In connection with early claims for the beneficial effect of the brew on the health of the female sex glands, our attention is immediately drawn to the aspartic acid and vitamin E contained in honey. And science tells us that honey also contains traces of estrogen, part of the group of female hormones that are produced by the ovaries that are responsible for female sexuality and development. In considering the hop plant we learn that it, too, contains appreciable amounts of estrogen!

Modern Love Potion

Honey-beer is rather troublesome to prepare according to ancient recipes, therefore herbalists suggest a simple tea made from hops and honey. Place one ounce of hops in a porcelain or Pyrex container. Pour one pint of boiling water over the hops,

---

[1]*Prevention,* May 1969.

cover and allow to stand for 15 minutes, then strain. The tea is taken half an hour before meals in wineglassful doses to which a spoonful of pure honey has been added. The cold infusion may be reheated as desired.

WHEAT GERM OIL FOR SEX HEALTH

Wheat germ oil is rich in vitamin E and other valuable substances. Research shows that this fine natural product can help boost a woman's femininity and a man's virility. The oil has been reported to induce ovulation in previously barren women and to increase the sperm count in previously sterile men.

Farmers have known, long before science got around to proving it, that vitamin E as contained in wheat germ oil is the fertility factor. They didn't call it vitamin E, they just used fresh stone-ground wheat (which contains the wheat germ) and fed it to their magnificent stallions and other animals for breeding purposes. Poultry men also kept insisting that fresh wheat fed to chickens resulted in greater egg production. Breeders of minks, foxes, and sheep reported on the value of wheat germ oil in aiding reproduction. This information was cited many years ago in an article entitled "Hormones from the Wheat Fields."

Dr. Shute of Canada, renowned for his work with vitamin E and heart disease, has also used the vitamin extensively for reproductive disorders. He reports that experiments conducted on lab animals which were given a diet totally lacking in natural foods containing vitamin E resulted in derangements of sex life. It produced gradual atrophy of certain generative organs, resulting in the inability to manufacture sperm and eventually in total sterility. However, before the male organs became completely atrophied, administration of natural vitamin E could restore some sperm activity.

Dr. Shute prescribes vitamin E obtained from wheat germ oil in cases of interrupted pregnancies or sterility in his own patients. When a man and wife come to him he suggests that the husband's semen be examined for the possibility of defective sperm. Most of his male patients, however, are reluctant to cooperate. Dr. Shute says, "This illustrates better than anything else one could say, perhaps, men's fixed belief that their wives are at fault when their marriages are barren, and their peculiar vanity in respect to their own potency."

His percentage resulting from the treatment of male sterility showed that vitamin E therapy used daily for two weeks increased the sperm count in 48% of the patients, helped 67% to produce only live sperms when they previously had a high proportion or all of their sperms dead, and produced all normal forms in 56% of the men who had abnormal sperms before treatment.

Dr. Shute also reported on the effective results in treating barren women with vitamin E. In a good number of cases conception took place within a few weeks to several months after vitamin E therapy.

Value of Vitamin E in Pregnancy

When loss of an unborn child occurs any time between conception and 16 weeks, it is called abortion, whereas miscarriage means loss of the fetus any time after 16 weeks. Dr. Shute recounts his use of vitamin E in 153 pregnancies. Of these, 122 were threatened abortions and 87 in danger of having a miscarriage. A large percentage of these patients having either considerable bleeding or severe pain were saved with the aid of vitamin E therapy. Eighty-six % of the threatened miscarriages and 60% of the threatened abortions were successfully treated with natural vitamin E, resulting in normal births.

In an article written in the *Ohio State Medical Journal,* Drs. Silbernagel and Patterson warn that any woman who threatens to abort is a candidate for some form of therapy. "Obviously prophylaxis [prevention] if available would be better management," these medical authors say, and add, "Such an approach has been made possible by the use of a concentrate of wheat germ oil." They report on a series of 825 patients treated with wheat germ oil and 1,975 patients who were not. Of those taking the oil, the majority began using the product between the third and sixteenth week of pregnancy, and 5% were taking it before conception. In this group only 3.7% aborted. Of the group untreated with the oil, 15% aborted. Toxemia was present in only 2.1% of those using the wheat germ oil, but in 10% of those who did not take the remedy.

Vitamin E—Mother's "Best Friend"

Here is an interesting letter which appeared in a national health magazine:[2]

> May I place another feather in vitamin E's cap? After having four babies in the same number of years my breasts were like those of a tired old woman. Though I do not believe the female body should be a sex symbol, I was somewhat unhappy over the situation as I'm quite young and very much in love with my wonderful husband. I began doses of 300 units of vitamin E daily for a different reason, however, in hopes it would relieve some of the pain and unsightliness of my varicose veins. What a pleasant surprise I was in for, because within two weeks my breasts became as high and firm as any young girl's! It appears that also my abdominal muscles have firmed and my inches in general have "evened themselves up" (my weight is normal). My varicose veins? It's early yet in the game but I've had to wear support stockings only twice this month. In the pre-vitamin E days I wore them daily to relieve the constant aching and swelling.

Wheat Germ Oil—Rich Source of B Complex

M. S. Biskind reports in a publication, *Vitamins and Hormones,* that he found a relation between nutritional deficiencies and an unbalance of sex hormones. In women, the unbalance showed up as menstrual difficulties, acne, and painful breasts; in men, as softening of the testes, enlarged breasts, sparse body hair, and loss of sexual vigor. Both sexes were threatened by sterility. Biskind wrote: "Treatment with vitamin B complex, especially in the form of dessicated whole liver, produced, in addition to the healing of the vitamin deficiency, rapid and dramatic improvement in the endocrine disturbances."

Raw wheat germ and wheat germ oil are also rich sources of the vitamin B complex.

---

[2]*Prevention,* December 1966.

The Difference Between Natural Vitamin E and Wheat Germ Oil

What is the difference between a natural vitamin E preparation and wheat germ oil? Vitamin E isolated from wheat germ oil is pure vitamin E and nothing else, and in greater concentration than you'd get it in the wheat germ oil. The oil however contains not only vitamin E but also many other valuable nutrients like protein, minerals, and all the B vitamins which are important for good health.

Highly Perishable

Because of its high perishability, wheat germ oil rapidly becomes rancid and as a result loses its effectiveness. In a number of cases treated with this therapy by Dr. Shute, disappointing results could not be explained until he found the patients were storing their wheat germ oil at warm room temperature. Dr. Shute reports that wheat germ oil in capsules or bulk, once opened, does not retain its potency much longer than eight weeks even when refrigerated.

For Best Results

It has been pointed out by other medical doctors that it is best to take wheat germ oil when the stomach is reasonably empty; that is, between meals. In this way you are making sure the oil does not mix with any rancid fat that you may have eaten at mealtime.

Another point to be noted in taking wheat germ oil is whether or not you are also using commercially prepared iron supplements. These completely nullify the beneficial effect of the wheat germ oil. Nutritionalists suggest that in the case of iron, which is necessary especially for pregnant women (to prevent anemia), liver is the answer to the problem as it is a food containing iron in its natural form, which does not destroy the good effects of wheat germ oil. For those who do not care for whole liver, powdered dessicated liver available in capsules can be used instead.

THE SEX MAGIC OF GINSENG

Ginseng, the "Number One" Chinese medicinal plant prized in the Orient as a cure for illness and as an elixir for "staying young," is also highly valued in the Far East as a sex rejuvenant. Its history shows that it was being used to pep up fading virility by Chinese men for thousands of years. According to reports coming from the Far East, men who have passed the spring and summer of their lives and use ginseng regularly are able to satisfy their romantic desires as though they were young again.

The late Dr. S. N. Chernych of San Francisco was convinced that the Chinese claim for the sex-invigorating power of the ancient wonder-root was true. He said, "Oriental healers are successfully curing patients of sexual impotence by the use of ginseng, and sexual impotence is one of the most difficult disorders. I can state from personal experience that the Oriental physicians have cured several men whom I and several other doctors tried to help."

Chinese healers insist that ginseng *does not stimulate* the sex glands into unnatural activity but that it is a *restorer* of the normally healthy sexual function that has become "weary."

Ginseng—a Strengthener of the Glandular System

The potency of ginseng as a sex improver has been confirmed by Russian scientists who have been studying the Oriental plant for a great many years. They have established that the root has a beneficial influence on the sex glands and other endocrine glands. And their findings show that the effects do not lead to premature exhaustion of the organism, for the herb is definitely not a strong stimulant. Russian reports agree with Chinese claims that ginseng acts by healthfully invigorating the physiological processes.

Note: Russian studies were conducted on the species of ginseng known botanically as *Panax schinseng,* and not on the American variety called *Panax quinquefolium.* The Chinese variety is imported from Korea and can be obtained from herb companies here in the United States.

How Ginseng Is Used

Ginseng's "sex magic" is not instantaneous. Those who have used the root faithfully over a period of time unanimously agree that its strengthening effect on the reproductive system is slow and gradual.

Powdered ginseng is available in bulk form and in capsules for do-it-yourselfers. The bulk powder can be used as a tea or added to juices. On the other hand there are those who prefer to do as the Chinese do—chew a small portion of the root every day.

ANOTHER OLD-WORLD SEX REJUVENATOR

FENUGREEK *(Trigonella foenum-graecum)*
Part Used: The seeds.

Fenugreek is a leguminous herb from one to two feet high, with pods two to three inches long, pointed, having ten to 20 seeds in them. The plant is native to the Eastern shores of the Mediteranean, but has been widely cultivated in many countries throughout the world. It is an important ingredient in chutney, a spicy meat condiment, and also in Oriental curry recipes for lamb, etc. An extract of the seeds is used with other aromatic substances to make artificial maple flavoring. In some countries the seeds are roasted and used as a substitute for coffee beans.

The botanical name, *foenum-graecum,* means "Greek hay." In the Mediterranean and Far East countries it was mixed with hay and fed to cattle as an animal sex and general health conditioner. Perhaps the ancients first got the idea of including the seeds as an article of food in their own personal diets after they noticed the marked improvement in the animals. Eventually, fenugreek seeds were also included in botanical listings or pharmacopoeias. They are classified medicinally as aphrodiasiac (sex stimulating), demulcent, diuretic, nutritive, tonic, and carminative for stomach gas.

Since ancient times fenugreek has been held in high repute as a tonic to the reproductive system. Pliny, the ancient Roman sage who wrote a lengthy discourse on spice remedies, and quoted many herbal and medical authorities, says that fenugreek has a beneficial effect on the generative (sex) organs. He regards it as an effective treatment for female disorders and claims that it is also helpful in cases of difficult labor in giving birth. To this day the Turkish maidens of Tunisia still prepare and eat a mixture of honey and powdered fenugreek seed to improve their feminine figures and sexy appearance.

Potent Factors in Fenugreek

Fenugreek seeds contain protein and, according to a report in *Biological Abstracts,* "new free amino acids," the building blocks of the human body. Another substance found in the seeds is *trigonelline,* which the authoritative U.S. Pharmacopeia describes as the methylbetaine of nicotinic acid—the pellagra preventive factor. (Pellagra is a serious disease, world wide, resulting from nutritional deficiencies.) The seeds also contain an aromatic oil similar in composition to cod-liver oil, which is so rich in vitamin D. In India the seeds are used effectively as a substitute for fish oil, rich in vitamins preventing pellagra and serious nervous disorders.

The oil contained in fenugreek seed could account for the plant's ancient reputation as a sex rejuvenator for the animal or man deficient in vitamins A and D. For the past 40 years the damaging effects on the male organs resulting from vitamin A deficiency in the diet has been under scientific study. Experiments on laboratory animals showed marked reduction or complete loss of sperm as a consequence of vitamin A shortage. Scientists of the Royal Veterinary and Agricultural College, Copenhagen, Denmark, reported on experiments in which boars were fed a diet low in vitamin A. On this diet the animals' sperm count dropped. Daily injections of vitamin A in dosages varying between 6,000 and 8,000 international units gradually restored the sperm count to normal.

Another possible sex-rejuvenating property contained in fenugreek is *trimethylamine.* Scientific studies show that it acts as a sex hormone in frogs, causing them to prepare for mating.

How Fenugreek Seeds Are Used

Fenugreek can be made into a tea by steeping one teaspoonful of the seeds in one cup of boiling water. However, since heat destroys the enzymes, the full benefit of the seeds' inherent properties are not obtained when the diluted tea form is used. For best possible results, herbalists suggest adding the seeds in powdered form to foods or juices. Or from eight to ten fenugreek seed tablets (procurable from herbal dealers or health food stores) can be used daily instead of drinking fenugreek tea.

DAMIANA–THE MEXICAN APHRODISIAC AND TONIC

Mexican Damiana *(Turnera diffusa),* commonly called damiana.

Part Used: Leaves and tops.

Damiana is a small mint-like plant bearing fragrant yellowish-white flowers. Its natural habitat is Mexico, Lower California, and Texas.

Damiana is classified in the Mexican pharmacopoeia as aphrodisiac, tonic, and diuretic. It has been scientifically accepted in that country as a reliable remedy in cases of sexual impotence, especially when due to over-indulgence. It is also prescribed for spermatorrhea (involuntary emissions) and for treating orchitis, a condition resulting in atrophy of the testicles. The plant is credited with producing a beneficial effect on the spinal cord, and some Mexican physicians employ it as a brain tonic. Nervous debility and exhaustion have also been treated with damiana.

Practicing medical herbalists in different countries agree on the Mexican classification of damiana's therapeutic action. In *Potter's Cyclopaedia of Botanical Drugs and Preparations* we read: "Damiana is very largely prescribed on account of its aphrodisiac qualities, and there is no doubt that it has a very great and generally beneficial action on the reproductive organs. It also acts as a tonic to the nervous system."

Steinmetz, in his monumental work *Materia Medica Vegetabilis,* lists damiana as follows: "The leaves are a stimulant in sexual weakness and a tonic to the nerves. The drug is esteemed for its aphrodisiac properties and its excellent effect on the reproductive organs. It overcomes exhaustion and cerebral lassitude, and a tendency to loss of power in the limbs. It is also diuretic." (A diuretic stimulates kidney action.)

How Damiana Is Used

Damiana is used as an infusion or in the form of a dry or fluid extract. Professor Maximino Martinez of Mexico says, "An infusion of damiana is prepared with a teaspoon of leaves to a cup of water, taken before breakfast. Fifty drops of the extract in sweetened water or wine may also be taken daily."

Some medical herbalists contend that damiana's power as a tonic for sexual debility (weakness) is increased when the plant is combined with other appropriate herbs. Yemm, for example, recommends a mixture of one ounce each of the fluid extracts of damiana, kola, and saw palmetto for "nervous and sexual debility." He recommends a small teaspoonful in a wineglass of water three times a day before meals, and advises that the diet be light and easily digestible.

CHAPTER SUMMARY

1. The use of herbs as "love potions" dates from antiquity. Just as plants have proved valuable in the development of modern medicines such as digitalis, ephedrine and many others, evidence is steadily accumulating that a number of the ancient folk tales about herbs as builders of sex health are based on medical fact.
2. The herbs and plant products mentioned in this chapter are not aphrodisiacs in the popular concept of the term; that is, they do not stimulate the sex organs into unnatural activity. They work by feeding the glands with the nutrients needed to restore normal, healthy functioning. Another important feature of herbs is that they supply the nutritional elements in a naturally wholesome form that the body can easily assimilate.
3. When considering the use of herbs to help you improve your sex capacities it is important to realize that the more properly balanced your diet is, the better the herbs will work.
4. Sexual inadequacies such as female frigidity, sterility, male impotence, premature ejaculation, can strain a marriage to the breaking point. Herbs and a sensible diet can play a real role in helping men and women to enjoy happier, fuller love lives.

2

How Herbs Can Help Restore
Youthful Digestive Powers

When the "Mayflower" landed on the bleak shores of Cape Cod on December 21, 1620, a total of 102 persons faced the onset of what was to be a long and extremely brutal winter. Malnutrition from weeks of vitamin-deficient sea diet left them in a weakened state, and the shortage of fats in their bodies exposed them to the paralyzing cold. Then came the revolting gangrene, sickening dysentery, and vile abscesses. Many died.

The courageous survivors clung desperately to the slim thread of life, and when at last they felt that the limits of human endurance had been reached the storms abated, the sky cleared, and they saw they were not alone. Animals, also lashed by hunger and the cruel elements, dotted the winter landscape. Fear of man had strangely deserted these wild creatures in their moment of desperation, and they were seen stripping bark from certain trees with their teeth. The settlers got the message. The strongest dragged themselves over the snow-covered slope, and with the aid of a boat hook ripped off slivers of the bark. This was quickly boiled to a thick gruel in the colony cauldron. New hope burst forth in desperate hearts as strength began to return. Colic disappeared, delicate stomachs and weak eyes grew stronger. Spreading the demulcent gruel on their ulcers, the settlers gave thanks for yet another miracle as sores healed. The virtues of slippery elm, the "Oohooska" tree of the Indians, had been discovered.

Modern Uses of Slippery Elm Bark

Today, finely powdered slippery elm bark is considered one of nature's finest demulcents, and is used for its ability to neutralize stomach acidity and to absorb foul gases. Its action is so gentle that it can be retained by a delicate stomach when other foods or even water is rejected. Among its other abilities, it aids the digestion of milk by separation of the casein particles. This can be considered of benefit to children, invalids, the aged, and to those with a touchy digestion. Because of its mucilaginous or "oozy" nature, its use assures an easy passage during the process of assimilation and elimination. It also acts as a buffer against irritation and inflammation of the mucous membranes.

On its own, the powdered bark of this tree is difficult to mix without forming lumps. For this reason the tea is prepared by adding two teaspoonfuls of the powder in a half-cup of cold water. This is placed in a container and shaken thoroughly. One pint of boiling water is then added and the mixture stirred.

The gruel is made by heating a half-pint of milk or water and sprinkling one teaspoonful of finely powdered slippery elm bark into the liquid. This is beaten thoroughly with an electric mixer or egg beater, then boiled until it thickens. Some prefer to beat up an egg with one teaspoonful of the powdered bark. Boiling milk is then poured over the mixture which is stirred and sweetened to taste.

Many preparations of slippery elm are sold on the market as bland and nutritious foods. In some cases the powdered bark is added to a base of barley malt and pre-cooked wheaten flour. An important feature of this finished product is that the mixture contains the active enzymes of malted barley which have the ability to convert cereal starches into soluble, and therefore more digestible, carbohydrates—maltose and dextrins.

CHRONIC INDIGESTION—A COMMON AILMENT

An estimated 30 million people in the United States suffer from chronic digestive disturbances. Eating too fast; food swallowed in large pieces; wrong food combinations; drinking too much fluid with meals; intolerance toward sugars, starches and fats; over-eating; swallowing air when eating; stress and emotional upset—these are among the many usual causes of indigestion. The common symptoms are heartburn, coated tongue, sour belchings, a heavy distressed feeling in the stomach after a meal, flatulence, a bad taste in the mouth, nausea, and sometimes difficult breathing and palpitation.

Of the acid-forming foods, meats, fish, and fowl head the list because (1) they contain considerable amounts of phosphorus and sulphur which are acid forming, and (2) they contain their own cellular wastes, such as uric acid for example, which were present in the blood and tissues at the time the animal was butchered. This second factor brings to mind one of the ancient Biblical rules of diet in which the eating of meat that has not been well drained of blood is prohibited.

Peanuts, lentils, eggs, cheese, and all cereals and grains rate close to meat in acid content.

HOW CERTAIN HERBS CAN HELP TONE UP THE STOMACH

Writings on the use of herbs as an aid for toning up the stomach take us back many centuries. In former times every home had its own herb garden, and the lady of the house always seemed to know just which herb was best for improving the appetite, and which one would relieve heartburn, gas, sour eructations, or nausea. These old remedies are still with us and are rapidly regaining their former popularity.

In the following list it will be noted that herbs used to improve digestibility are recognized culinary herbs. The whole subject of herbs in cookery has recently come into the limelight and more and more recipes are appearing in women's magazines. Yet most people think of culinary herbs solely in terms of flavor, not realizing that their original purpose was therapeutic. When the ancients began adding more meat and heavy rich foods to their diet they found they were getting sick, so they conceived the idea of taking their medicine with their food and included herbs such as ginger, fennel, anise, sage, or mint to help prevent indigestion. *Mint* added to peas, for example, helps correct the tendency of peas to produce gas. And the custom of serving mint sauce with lamb is not merely a matter of taste; young meat is more difficult to digest, and the mint serves to prevent it from "disagreeing." *Marjoram,* another popular culinary herb, was also employed mainly as a digestive aid. An old herb book states: "Sweet marjoram is chiefly used as a condiment in cooking, to diminish by its excitant qualities the heaviness of pork, goose, and other foods."

The American Indians also fully recognized the true purpose of culinary herbs and combined them with food to improve digestibility. The flavor factor was secondary.

Unless otherwise directed, the procedure in each of the following remedies is generally the same as for preparing your ordinary tea: boiling water is poured over the leaves, or if a tea is made from the seeds or root, it is generally boiled for about ten or 15 minutes.

ANGELICA *(Angelica archangelica)*

Synonyms: Garden angelica, archangelica, holy herb.
Part Used: Leaves, stems, roots, seeds.

It is said that the name *angelica* was given to this plant because it blossoms on the archangel St. Michael's Day. Another version has it that the herb was so named during the Middle Ages when a devout man dreamed that St. Michael appeared and told him the plant was a cure for the dreaded plague. In the contemporary descriptions of those times one can find repeated references to the belief that anyone who kept a piece of angelica root in his mouth all day would be immune from contagious disease. The plant was also endowed with magic powers and used as a charm against witchcraft and the evil eye.

Angelica has always been a popular flavoring agent, and a kitchen medicine for indigestion. In some countries the stalks are candied, the roots roasted, and the leaves prepared and eaten like spinach. The seeds or roots used as a tea is an old-time favorite for relieving gas pains.

Dr. Vogel of Switzerland says that the fresh plant extract of angelica has an excellent effect on the digestion; on irritation of the gastric mucous membrane; on loss of appetite; and also on stomach cramps.[1] He advises ten drops in water to be taken three times a day, half an hour before meals. Dr. Vogel mentions that the seeds also may be used, and gives the recipe for genuine Angelica Liqueur, "Vespetro." Two ounces of Angelica seeds, ¼ ounce of anise seeds, ¼ ounce of fennel seeds, and approximately 1/5 ounce of coriander seeds are ground together in a seed mill. Eight fluid ounces of pure drinkable alcohol (not rubbing alcohol) is added and the preparation allowed to stand for eight days. It is then strained through muslin and mixed with a solution of one pound of sugar (preferably grape sugar) dissolved in two and a half pints of water.

Of this recipe Dr. Vogel says, "There is no better or more pleasant remedy for digestive troubles or flatulence." He invites us to imagine a monastery of olden times: "There the monks enjoy a glass of the golden drink before appearing for duty in the mornings; and late in the evening, a guest arriving with perhaps a chilled or troublesome stomach, would be given a glass of 'Vespetro,' a small sip of which would have a quicker and better effect than the chemical tablet of today."

ANISE *(Pimpinella anisum)*

Part Used: Leaves, seeds.

Anise is of Eastern origin but is now cultivated in many parts of the world. It has an ancient reputation as a carminative, stomachic, expectorant, and flavoring agent. Several centuries ago the Romans and Greeks used anise in relishes, seasonings, sauces, and wines (just as we do today). The seeds were chewed as a breath sweetener and to stimulate the appetite. The Romans served a wedding cake strongly flavored with anise seeds to help prevent indigestion caused by overeating at the marriage banquet. From this ancient practice came the tradition of baking special cakes for weddings. Gerard, an early herbalist, recommended anise seeds as "good against belchings and upbrading of the stomacke."

Anise is still considered a good domestic remedy for preventing gas and fermentation in the stomach and bowels if a tea is brewed from the seeds and taken warm.

---

[1]Dr. h.c. A. Vogel, *The Nature Doctor* (Teufen AR Switzerland: Bioforce-Verlag, 1960), p. 181.

FENNEL *(Foeniculum vulgare)*

Synonyms: Sweet fennel.
Part Used: Leaves, herb, seeds.

Fennel, "the friend of the stomach," has been used since earliest times as a culinary herb and medicine. It is reputed to have a soothing effect on the mucous membrane and to be wonderfully effective in helping people bothered with excessive belching and flatulence. There are also recommendations for its use in cookery as an aid in the digestion of fish, beans, peas, cheese, and cabbage.

Amerigo Vespucci, for whom America was named, often mentions fennel in an account to a grandee of Florence. He stated, "For after the care and thought your affairs demand, my letter may afford you some little pleasure, just as fennel gives a better flavor to the food one has eaten and helps digestion."

In Grandma's time the people used a light, bland diet, and drank four or five cups of pleasant-tasting fennel seed tea a day for several days following an upset stomach or stomach distress. One or two teaspoonfuls of the warm tea was given to infants for the relief of colic. The seeds were also employed to check griping tendencies of laxatives or purgatives.

In Italy, the use of the dwarf variety of fennel *(F. dulce)* called *finocchio* dates from the days of the early Romans when gladiators mixed the herb with their food, claiming that it gave them strength. Today, fennel is still best known to people of Italian descent, and Italy is its greatest stronghold. It is maintained that foods difficult to digest such as rich and oily fish give no trouble if fennel sauce is served with them.

Fennel Sauce. To prepare the sauce, strip the fennel from the stalks, chop into small pieces, and simmer in boiling water for about ten minutes. Strain and add to hot melted butter.

Fennel Tea. Fennel tea is made by placing two teaspoonfuls of the seed into a half-cup of boiling water. Boil one minute, cover the vessel to retain the aromatic oil, strain and allow to become just warm.

GINGER *(Zingiber officinale)*

Part Used: Root.

Ginger is an ancient perennial herb native to Asia. It is produced commercially in Jamaica, Africa, Japan, China, India, and the Dutch East Indies; the best is reputed to be that of Jamaica.

Some professional Chinese cooks keep a small piece of ginger root in their mouth to prevent nausea from prolonged exposure to cooking odors. In China, the poorer classes test food by tossing a slice of fresh ginger into their cooking pot. They claim that if the root turns a dark color the food is bad.

Chinese Ginger Recipe for Healthful Digestion

Ginger holds a high position in Chinese materia medica. Following is a secret Chinese formula reputed to be excellent for restoring strength to the stomach and promoting a healthy digestion:

Step 1. Put one-half cup of white rice in a flat bowl. Pour in enough water to barely cover the rice. Let stand overnight so that the water may be completely absorbed by the rice. In the morning if there is any water still standing in the bowl, drain it off. Put the rice in a dry frying pan and gradually heat until the pan is very hot. Use a spatula and keep turning the rice slowly so it doesn't burn. When the rice is parched dry and golden brown put it in a glass jar and cap tightly against moisture.

Step 2. Bring one cup of water to a boil; add one teaspoon of the parched rice and a small piece of ginger root. Boil for one minute, then turn off the burner and let stand for five minutes. Strain. Take one teacupful, once or twice a day.

The Chinese claim this remedy is especially good during the cold weather as it has a warming and comforting effect on the stomach and is felt throughout the entire system.

An English Doctor's Ginger Formula for Healthful Digestion

Here is a remedy in which ginger is blended with other herbs to help tone up the stomach. H. Darwent, M.N.I.M.H., of England, says: "I have used this formula in my practice for years and it has always given splendid results."

Centaury . . . . ½ oz.
Raspberry leaves . . . . . . ½ oz.
Agrimony . . . . ½ oz.
Dandelion leaves . . . . . . ½ oz.
Wormwood . . . . ½ oz.
Ginger root . . . . ¼ oz.
Senna . . . . ¼ oz.

(If an aperient [laxative] is not required, leave out the senna.)

Directions: Mix well and put half in two pints of cold water, bring to the boil and simmer for 15 minutes. Strain when cold and take half a teacupful before meals. Children can take *half the dose.*

Gastritis, nervous, acid or fermentive dyspepsia and catarrh of the stomach are similar stomach troubles which usually respond well to the above treatment.[2]

OKRA *(Hibiscus esculentus)*

Part Used: The pods.

Due to its mucilaginous (or viscous) and bland nature, okra is highly regarded as a demulcent food. Demulcents are prized for their protective or coating-like properties and are used internally to allay irritation of membranes. Okra also provides valuable minerals. U.S. Government Bulletin No. 232 states: "Okra is valued in the diet, chiefly because of the nutritionally important minerals it contains."

Powdered okra may be taken with water, or with other bland foods such as milk and broths. It is a popular ingredient in gumbo soup and Creole dishes.

Powdered Okra for Stomach Ulcers

Sufferers from stomach ulcers will be interested in the following report by Dr. Herman N. Bundesen:

"It was observed by a certain doctor that a patient who had mucous colitis, a disorder in which there are alternating attacks of constipation and diarrhea, was improved by using a large amount of . . . okra . . . . This observation led Dr. J. Meyer of Chicago and his co-workers to make a study of okra.

---

[2]*Health from Herbs,* May-June 1967, p. 91.

"They used a dry powdered okra in treating ulcer of the stomach and first part of the intestine. This okra is a light yellow-green color and has a fairly pleasant taste. When mixed with water, the powder becomes thick. However, the powdered okra was given to the patients in the form of a tablet or capsule.

"Seventeen persons with ulcer of the stomach or the first part of the intestines were given powdered okra as the only form of treatment for their condition. The diagnosis was made in each case by means of X-ray. All of the patients were having symptoms of ulcer of the stomach or first part of the intestine at the time the treatment was started.

"Of the seventeen patients who were treated, fourteen obtained immediate relief from their symptoms with the powdered okra treatment. One individual had no relief for three days after starting the okra treatment, but on the fifth day his symptoms did disappear.

"Evidently then the powdered okra does give quick relief from the symptoms of ulcer. . . ."

In reference to the study mentioned above, another American physician, Dr. Evans, had this to say: "Our old friend okra seems on the point of assuming new duties and responsibilities. The new job it is taking on is that of relieving the discomfort of ulcer of the stomach. It threatens to push bicarbonate of soda and mucin out of their chief employment as a medicine.

"A few years ago it occurred to some physicians that if 'gooey' stuff from animal sources was of service in treating the pain and discomfort of stomach ulcer, similar material of vegetable origin might have the same effect and yet be more pleasant to take . . . . Then it was recalled that okra . . . because of some mucilaginous content . . .might be worthy of trial.

"Different groups have been using it for several months. Drs. J. Meyer, E. E. Seidmon and H. Necheles published a report of seventeen cases. The results obtained were quite as good as those given by any other treatment.

"As a rule, the users like to chew the okra tablets. The treatment was popular both on its own account and also because it was a means of escape from more unpleasant 'goos.' It was found taking okra powder not only eased the discomfort but also caused the stomach to empty more promptly. . . . ."

PAPAYA *(Carica papaya)*

Part Used: The fruit.

Centuries ago natives of the tropics found they could eat exceptionally heavy meals of fish and meat without any apparent stomach distress if the meal was followed by a dessert of papaya. Modern research has shown that this tropical melon-like fruit contains a powerful protein-digesting enzyme called *papain* which greatly resembles pepsin, the natural digestive enzyme found in the stomach. Papain extracted from the unripe papaya melon is so powerful that five grains of the white crystalline powder are said to digest a pint of milk in half an hour.

The natural papain enzyme is made into tablets and sold as an aid to digestion. The tablet acts on acid, alkaline, or neutral conditions without being destroyed by intestinal juices. It is considered especially valuable as an aid to normal digestion of protein in the stomach.

Proteins in nutrition are the basic building material of every cell in the body. Energy, ability to withstand "wear and tear," and muscle-building depend upon the proteins we get in our food. But proteins must be liquified and digested before they can pass their benefits into the bloodstream. Incomplete digestion often leads to constipation and other distressing conditions.

The best sources of protein are meat, fish, cheese, eggs, poultry, brewer's yeast, soy beans, wheat germ, and some varieties of nuts. Protein foods decompose more rapidly than other foods, and the longer they are retained in the intestinal tract the more likely they are to cause a toxic condition. In a matter of hours decomposed protein foods cause sulphurated hydrogen—a polite term for putrid gases, ensuing bloat, bad mouth taste, and foul breath.

Papaya enzyme tablets are especially effective upon meat, and increases its utilization by making it more assimilable. They also improve the utilization of fats, starches; and carbohydrates as well as the protein contained in plant foods such as peas, beans, lentils, nuts, and cereals. The tablets also assist the digestion of meals cooked in grease or fats.

With the use of papaya enzyme tablets you can help nature digest valuable protein foods and in this way help protect yourself against protein indigestion—gas, heartburn, and sour stomach. One woman said, "I am so happy since I found out about papaya tablets. I was always filled with gas—even water caused gas. This has disappeared like magic since taking them." In another case: There was a man plagued with dyspepsia, much to the distress of his wife. She complained, "He would clutch his middle and issue a series of little moans like owls wailing among the ruins of some buried city. Papain killed all the owls and now he's fairly hooting for his fish and chips."[3]

PEPPERMINT *(Mentha piperita)*

Synonyms: Lammint, Brandy Mint.
Part Used: The herb.

Peppermint tea is a valuable old-time beverage which tends to relieve stomach gas, flatulence, and resultant distresses. It is comforting to the stomach and agreeable to the system. As a harmless caffeine-free beverage it will not cause restlessness or keep you awake nights. Palatable, aromatic and refreshing, it can be taken as a wholesome tisane by every member of the family. For young children, one or two tablespoonfuls of the tea can be sweetened with honey.

HERBAL TREATMENT FOR GASTRITIS

Following is an excerpt from an article written by Arthur C. Hyde, M.N.I.M.H., a practicing medical herbalist of England.[4]

Catarrhal conditions of the digestive tract may cause only mild discomfort from time to time, or may be extremely severe. Gastritis means catarrh of the stomach itself, and is often associated with catarrh in the food pipe and the first portion of the small intestine. Catarrh of the small bowel is called enteritis, while that in the large bowel is termed colitis. As the digestive tract is one complete system, catarrh of any part affects, directly or indirectly, the other areas, quite apart from its effect on the rest of the body systems.

There are two main types of gastritis, acute and chronic. This grouping generally holds true for catarrh of the other parts of the digestive system, the acute form being caused by some specific irritant or an allergy. The commonest irritants met with are alcohol,

---

[3] *Grace,* Summer, 1969.
[4] *Health from Herbs,* May-June 1967, p. 92-3.

strong tea and coffee, tobacco and many modern drugs, notably pain-killers. Chronic digestive catarrh may be of several forms, but the symptoms and treatment are very similar in each case. The swallowing of infected mucus produced during a head cold or influenza may also cause gastritis.

How a Long-Standing Case of Stomach Trouble Was Handled

The patient, a gentleman in his forties, holding a responsible position in business, described his symptoms as heartburn and nausea after meals, coupled with sharp pains in the stomach region, and a feeling of being bloated following even a fairly light meal. This had been happening for over five years, and all treatment had so far proved ineffectual. Upon examination, I found that there was an area of discomfort in the stomach region, and a sensation of nausea upon pressure; there was also quite appreciable flatulence in the stomach, causing some distension. Because the pains were felt at differing intervals after taking food, and with the knowledge that a recent X-ray had shown nothing structurally abnormal, I was able to exclude ulcers, and completing my investigation, to arrive at a diagnosis of chronic gastritis. The patient smoked up to twenty cigarettes a day, liked to take whiskey in fairly large doses, and was fond of very strong tea.

Correct diet is most important in clearing any condition of illness, especially of the digestive system. Also, adequate rest and freedom from anxiety are essential if a full return to health is to be achieved. I advised care not to overtax mental and nervous resources, to avoid lifting heavy weights, and to keep warm, because strain and chilling only aggravate the trouble. The dietary regimen was based upon the following:

Avoid acid foods—such as vinegar and pickles; irritant foods—such as pepper, spices, alcohol, strong tea and coffee; roughage—such as peas and beans, crusts, peels and skins of fruit, and raw or partially cooked green vegetables; all dried foods. Take bland foods—such as slippery elm, milk, and foods prepared in milk, white meats (chicken and fish), vegetables cooked and sieved, and weak tea. All drink and solid food to be taken warm, not hot.

The patient agreed to adhere to the diet, and to try to stop smoking. This course of action together with herbal medicine helped the gentleman to regain his health and strength in a matter of months, and all symptoms have now disappeared.

Herbal Treatment

The medicine prescribed in this case, for gastritis, included remedies to regulate the production of stomach acid, by relieving the nervous tension, together with remedies to sooth the mucous lining of the digestive tract, and to help dry up excessive secretions.

Gastritis, enteritis, and catarrh of the food pipe respond well to the following herbal remedies:

> Chamomile flowers
> Meadowsweet herb
> Black Horehound herb
> Cranesbill herb
> Marshmallow root
> Comfrey leaves and root

In gastritis an infusion of:

Chamomile flowers	2 drachms
Meadowsweet herb	1 oz.
Marshmallow root	½ oz.
Black Horehound herb	½ oz.

in 1 pint of boiling water may be taken, 2-4 teaspoonfuls in the same quantity of hot water, one-half hour before meals.

BITTERS FOR BETTER DIGESTION

The custom of employing bitters as a stomach tonic is age-old. Romans, notorious for their overindulgences, believed bitters were necessary with food. The Indians also appreciated the natural bitter of herbs, vegetables, and fruits. Early explorers found the natives of South America eating potatoes but said that the tubers were too bitter for their own taste. It was only after ages of cultivation by the white man that the common potato has become large, pulpous, and almost tasteless.

Today, bitters are still highly valued by many people. In Iceland, Lapland, and Greenland, bread and beverages are made of bitterish Iceland moss; bitter herbs are also added to wines, liquors and beer. In other nations some people gather the bitter leaves of the wild dandelion early in the spring and use them in salads.

Among the Germans, gentian is a highly prized bitter herb. It is reputed to be a powerful tonic which strengthens the digestion and improves the appetite to a remarkable degree. In the last century Father Kneipp, the renowned herbalist and water healer, wrote:

"Before all, I advise you to prepare an extract of gentian. The gentian roots are for this purpose well dried, cut small, then put into bottles with brandy or spirit. (Steep for one week, then strain.)

"This extract is one of the best stomachics. Put six to eight tablespoonfuls of water into a glass, and pour in 20 to 30 drops of extract; take this mixture daily for some time. The good digestion will soon be indicated by a no less good appetite. If the food is felt to lie heavy in the stomach, and is troublesome, a little cordial made with a teaspoonful of extract in half a glass of water will soon stop the disorder.

"Gentian is likewise very good for cramp in the stomach. When after a long journey during which for days together eating fares badly and drinking still worse, people arrive at their destination dead tired and almost ill, a tiny bottle of gentian tincture taken in drops on sugar will render excellent service.

"Nausea and attacks of faintness are removed by taking a teaspoonful of tincture in water; it warms, enlivens, and brings body and mind to peace again."

Favorite Bitter Tonic of the American Indians

Golden seal *(Hydrastis canadensis)* was highly regarded by the Cherokee Indians as a bitter tonic and also as an external remedy for various complaints. Early writers credited the Cherokees with introducing the plant to the settlers. Later, the medical profession took an interest in the herb and many reports of its use began to appear in medical writings. In reference to golden seal, Hand *(House Surgeon,* 1820) wrote, "It may be given in form of powder or strong tea made by boiling, in indigestion . . . ." *The Thomsonian Recorder,* 1833, reviewed the medical uses of golden seal described by others and added, "It admirably relieves stomach oppression, nausea, and heartburn." It was also stated to be a good remedy "for the peculiar sickness attendant in females during their periods of utero-gestation, called morning sickness."

Golden seal is pleasantly bitter and somewhat pungent to the taste. Dr. Ellingwood wrote: "Its widest range of action is upon the stomach." And in the opinion of Curtis, golden seal should constitute an ingredient in bitters, "as it will often remove heaviness after eating."

In a modern British volume on botanical drugs,[5] golden seal is cited as a valuable remedy in disordered states of the digestive system: "As a general bitter tonic it is applicable to debilitated conditions of mucous tissues. As a remedy for various gastric disorders it takes a leading place, acting very beneficially in acute inflammatory conditions. It will be found of value in all cases of dyspepsia, biliousness, and debility of the system."

Mattson suggests one teaspoon of golden seal powder steeped in one-half cup of hot water. It may be sweetened to make it more palatable. Putting the powder in capsules which are then swallowed with a little water is another popular method of using golden seal.

Recipe for Golden Seal Spice Bitters[6]

Steep in sherry wine or brandy equal parts of dried orange peel, prickly ash and golden seal root. Take in small doses before meals after mixture has been allowed to steep a week or ten days. Botanicals may be strained off or allowed to remain in liquor.

Yarrow—a Specific for Nausea

Bitter herbs are very important to mountaineers of Switzerland, and no chalet is without its store of botanicals to brew a stomach cordial or appetite tonic. Schafgarbe (yarrow) is used by the Swiss as a bitter tea and highly revered among them.

Yarrow *(Achillea millefolium)* was well known to the American Indians who applied it externally on bruises, cuts, sores, etc., and used it as a tea for weak and disordered stomachs. The colonists employed it as a bitter. Dr. Clapp called the herb a mild astringent, the leaves being more potent than the blossoms, and the American species more active than the European. It was used by the frontier doctors in diarrhoea, mild forms of bleeding, and dyspepsia.

[5]R. C. Wren, *Potter's New Cyclopaedia of Botanical Drugs and Preparations,* (Sir Isaac Pitman & Sons Ltd., London) 7th ed. 1956.

[6]*Herbalist Almanac,* 1966, Indiana Botanic Gardens.

In modern herbals we find yarrow tea listed as a specific against nausea, and cited as a reliable bitter tonic, "both stimulating the appetite and toning the organs of digestion." One or two cups of tea made from the leaves or blossoms is reputed to stop nausea within minutes.

Yarrow yields a volatile oil containing *azulene,* and *achilleine,* a glyco-alkaloid; also gum, tannin, resin, chlorides of calcium and potassium, and various salts such as nitrates, malates, and phosphorus.

SELECTED HERBAL REMEDIES AS REPORTED IN USAGE FOR VARIOUS STOMACH TROUBLES

Nervous Stomach

1. Cinnamon tea offers helpful moments of relaxation for the stomach upset by the tension and strain of modern living.
2. Balm or spearmint tea are popular remedies for nervous dyspepsia.

Acid Condition

1. According to a Chinese materia medica, a tea made from cardamom seeds will counteract acidity of the stomach.
2. English herbalists recommend an infusion of meadowsweet or black horehound to relieve acidity.

Gas Pains

1. An infusion made from catnip is a popular old-fashioned remedy for flatulence or colic in children and the aged. It may be sweetened to taste, and should be taken warm.
2. Oil of caraway is cited as an excellent carminative for excessive gas in the stomach or bowels. One or two drops of the oil may be taken on a small lump of sugar.

Digestion Aid

Fennel seed or a few dried leaves of rosemary steeped in olive oil makes a tasty dressing which greatly assists the digestibility of raw vegetable salads and also helps to prevent the formation of gas.

Distaste for Food

1. A pinch of ground ginger added to chamomile tea is a favorite domestic remedy for loss of appetite or distaste for food. Herbalists say that children may be given the warm tea in teaspoonful doses.
2. Another remedy reputed to aid digestion and stimulate the appetite consists of five drops of oil of lavender mixed with approximately half to one teaspoonful of honey, taken twice a day.

Liquor Abuses

1. Many people troubled with upset stomach as a result of excessive drinking have benefited considerably by taking one or two cups of ginger tea for breakfast.
2. Ellingwood's *Materia Medica Therapeutica and Pharmacognosy* states that a tea of "horsemint is efficient in the control of vomiting due to exhaustion, persistent nausea with flatulence, or vomiting of alcoholics in whom it will impart a temporary tone to the stomach."
3. This simple tip for "hangover" was offered by an old family recipe book: "The infusion of cloves may be advantageously given in dyspepsia, particularly when it arises from the abuse of ardent spirits."
4. A decoction of a little agar-agar sweetened to taste is recommended as a valuable demulcent, especially for heavy drinkers.

CHAPTER SUMMARY

1. Various culinary herbs listed here help to relieve indigestion and tone the stomach.
2. Symptoms of indigestion may appear as heartburn, coated tongue, gas pains, headache, loss of appetite, nausea, vomiting,

sour eructations, foul breath, bad taste in the mouth, and sometimes palpitations and difficult breathing.

3. Botanicals provided by nature not only bring about the desired results in digestive disorders but also work in a very gentle manner.

4. How specific culinary herbs, combined with certain foods, help prevent indigestion is discussed.

5. The use of herbal bitters, homemade teas and various herbal mixtures to counteract stomach acidity, nausea, and nervous indigestion is described in detail.

3

How Herbs Can Help
Strengthen Your Vision

Years ago a physician residing in Paris became renowned for his successful treatment of certain conditions affecting the eyes. His fame quickly spread throughout the city as word got around that many of his patients were able to discard their eye glasses after taking his treatment.

The majority of cases treated by the French medic involved some form of eye inflammation; conditions such as blepharitis and conjunctivitis were commonplace. The remedy he prescribed was a simple herb called eyebright *(Euphrasia officinalis)*. This was generally used in the form of an eye lotion; however, in some instances it was also taken internally as a tea.

Famed for Centuries as an Eye Remedy

For centuries, the herb eyebright has been regarded as a specific remedy for tired, inflamed, watering eyes. And it is interesting to note that in most European languages the plant's value as an eye medicine is indicated in its name. For example, in French it is called *casse-lunettes,* "breaker of spectacles"; the Italians call it *luminella,* "light for the eyes"; and the Germans, *Augentrost,* "consolation to the eyes."

As early as the 14th century the beneficial effects of eyebright on faulty vision were recognized and the plant described as the source of "a precious water to clear a man's sight." In the 17th century, Culpeper, the renowned English herbalist, said of eyebright: "Indeed it has a powerful effect to help and restore sight decayed through age."

MODERN USES OF EYEBRIGHT HERB

Today eyebright still enjoys its reputation as a remedy for certain problems affecting the vision. Dr. Dorothy Shepherd, for example, cites many of her case histories where prolonged use of eyebright lotion produced successful results in various eye conditions. (She also found the herb to be of value in the treatment of measles.)

Eyebright—a Sight for Sore Eyes

Dr. Jon Evans of England writes:[1]

The plant [eyebright] has a specific action on the mucous lining of the eyes, the nose, and uppermost parts of the throat as far as the windpipe. Its action on the lachrymal structures [causing tears to flow] of the eyes is the prime reason for its use in cases of measles because it prevents the eyes from being injured.

As the common name of the plant would imply, its influence is, in the main, associated with eye conditions. For the treatment of conjunctivitis I know of nothing more effective than the use of a lotion made from this wonderful remedy. The misery produced by conjunctivitis is only too well known, exuding white matter which often causes the eyelids to stick together with a smarting and almost unbearable irritation.

The proportions used for the lotion are exactly as those indicated for the infusion, one ounce of the whole dried herb to one pint of boiling water. The eyes should be bathed three to four times a day. The liquid should be well strained; if the infusion is allowed to stand for a half hour or so the particles of the herb will settle at the bottom of the jug.[2] When the eyes are very painful the lotion should be warmed before using it. The fresh plant tincture may be used but as this is considerably stronger be sure to use only three drops in a tablespoonful of boiled water [allow to cool before using]; a stronger solution may make the eyes smart. Whichever method you use, the eyebath should be freshly filled for each eye.

---

[1]*Health from Herbs,* September-October 1969.

[2]Herbal infusions may be strained by filtering through absorbent cotton.

Prevention and Maintenance

The following information on the use of eyebright is from *Acta Phytotherapeutica,* a Dutch scientific journal on botanical medicine.[3]

> Every student of herbs knows the uses of *Euphrasia officinalis* or eyebright. It is the main herb for protecting and maintaining the health of the eye. It acts as an internal medicine for the constitutional tendency to eye weakness in fluid extract form at the dosage of ten drops three times daily or an infusion of the crude cut herb, one ounce to one pint of water in wineglass doses three times daily.

The journal reports that an even more effective method is a local application of a lotion "made from three drops of fluid extract of Euphrasia in an eyebathful of cold water." The eyes are bathed morning and night.

> For the treatment of inflammation of the eyelids or the tendency to mucus accumulations in the eyes and redness of the rims of the eyelids, bathing with *Euphrasia* eye lotion should be supplemented by the addition of one drop of fluid extract of *Hydrastis canadensis* [golden seal] in an eyebath of the lotion.

Eyebright and Rosewater

William Smith, D.O., F.N.I.M.H., M.D.N.O.A., suggests a combination of a tincture of eyebright added to rose water, "about the strength of one of the former to 20 parts of the latter," as an eye bath for simple conditions of inflamed eyes. "Use several times daily."

A Remarkable Case History of Eye Inflammation Healing

A leading homeopathic journal cited an impressive case history where Euphrasia (eyebright) brought about marked improvement in a distressing eye condition.

A woman had a fair-sized cyst on the right lower eyelid, the result of chronic conjunctivitis. Over the years three or four cysts had been surgically removed and she dreaded the thought of another operation. Both eyes were inflamed and heavy-looking. In addition to the cyst, the right eye was swollen, lumpy, and "wept" when she was out of doors.

---

[3]Vol. XII, No.9, 1965, Amsterdam, Netherlands.

One day, during a casual conversation, a man noticed the woman's eye condition and suggested that she visit a homeopathic pharmacy. She took up the suggestion and was given this prescription: "Euphrasia 6 in tablets, with a recommended dose of two tablets hourly for a day, and then three times daily, and some Euphrasia mother tincture [homeopathic], one drop to be used in an eyebath of water once or twice daily."

Two weeks after she began using the Euphrasia tablets and tincture, both her eyes were clear and almost free from inflammation. The swelling of the right eye was entirely gone, and the cyst reduced in size.

The woman went back to her eye specialist, who was astonished to see her improved condition. He said he had never heard of Euphrasia, but told her to continue the treatment for another month, then come back and see him again.

Following her doctor's instructions she purchased a month's supply of the tablets and tincture. A week later the cyst was hardly larger than a pimple, and there was only a very faint trace of inflammation on the eyelid. At the end of the month, she reported that her specialist confirmed undoubted and marked improvement. He advised that she continue with the treatment which was obviously producing such excellent results.

Note: In homeopathic medicine, the number which directly follows the name of the remedy, for example Euphrasia 6, refers to the potency.

THE IMPORTANCE OF VITAMIN A TO YOUR EYES

Centuries ago herbalists wrote that parsley was highly beneficial for the health of the eyes. Today, modern nutritionalists tell us that this humble herb is extremely rich in vitamins A and C, with appreciable amounts of the vitamin B factors. Parsley also contains calcium, iron, phosphorus, manganese, and potassium.

Nightblindness—poor vision in dim illumination—is successfully treated with vitamin A. Normal eyes have a high content of vitamin C, so apparently this nutrient is very important to the health of the eyes (cataract patients have been found lacking in vitamin C). Calcium is needed for the eye muscles and for the fluid of the eye. The *American Journal of Ophthalmology*[4] suggests that myopia or nearsightedness is due to calcium and vitamin A deficiency.

In view of these facts we realize that the early herbalists were correct in their claims for parsley as a health fortifying herb for the eyes even though they knew nothing whatever of the existence of vitamins and minerals.

How Vitamin A Deficiency Affects the Eyes

Nightblindness, from which some ten million Americans suffer, is one of the earliest signs of vitamin A deficiency. With a mild deficiency a person sees more effectively in daylight than at night, and may experience eye fatigue after reading or watching TV, for example. If the lack is greater he may suffer a painful sensation in the eyes after long use, visual fatigue, nervousness, and headaches. When the shortage is severe, burning, itching, inflamed eyelids, and eye strain are experienced; sores or ulcers may sometimes appear on the eyes, and mucus may accumulate in the corners. A serious deficiency may be accompanied by scotomata—dark spots in the field of vision; or it is sometimes accompanied by dryness of the eye tissues and a gritty feeling as though grains of sand were on the eyeball *(xerophthalmia)*. If the dryness continues, the cornea softens and becomes dull, gray, and cloudy *(keratomalacia)*.

People lacking in vitamin A not only complain of difficulty in seeing well at night but also find that their eyes are extremely sensitive to light, such as the bright reflection from snow or the glare from automobile headlights and TV screens. The reason for this sensitivity is that prolonged exposure to bright light destroys vitamin A in the eyes. Bookkeepers, typists and stenographers who face the glare from white paper, or persons who spend much time sewing, reading, or studying under bright light, and people living on beaches or deserts where the sunlight is reflected by the sand are losing their vitamin A.

During the Second World War, American paratroopers were finally required to take the important eye vitamin when it was learned that the Japanese could spot our soldiers landing in the night before our paratroopers could see the Japanese.

---

[4] May 1950.

Approved Therapeutic Doses of Vitamin A

The following therapeutic doses of vitamin A have been approved by the Council on Pharmacy and Chemistry of the American Medical Association:

For prolonged or chronic deficiency, 25,000 units three times daily; for general treatment, 25,000 units twice daily for two months. Single doses larger than 25,000 units have not been approved.

Plant Sources of Vitamin A

With so many herbs and foods rich in vitamin A it is foolish to allow oneself to contract a deficiency that will result in eye trouble. So don't toss aside that decorative sprig of parsley on your plate. Eat a good amount every day. One-half cup of fresh chopped parsley contains approximately 8000 units of vitamin A, therefore the herb in large enough quantity in the diet can well provide enough of this precious vitamin to correct or prevent the condition of nightblindness and certain other visual difficulties.

Here is a brief list of other plant foods rich in vitamin A:

½ cup of cooked chard leaves contains 15,000 units vitamin A
½ cup of cooked dandelion leaves contains 20,000 units vitamin A
½ cup of cooked beet greens contains 22,000 units vitamin A
5 stalks of endive contains 7,500 units vitamin A
½ cup lamb's quarters herb contains 19,000 units vitamin A
1 medium sized sweet potato contains 3,600 units vitamin A
1 medium sized yam contains 5,000 units vitamin A

SUNFLOWER SEEDS—THE BETWEEN-MEAL SNACK FOR BETTER VISION

For snacking between meals you won't find anything more tasty or healthful for general vision than sunflower seeds. They contain all the important nutrients that benefit the eyes. In an issue of *Prevention* magazine, Mr. J. I. Rodale wrote:[5]

---

[5]March 1966.

My eyes are not my strongest point. In the winter I would have trouble in walking on snow-blanketed roads. Before I became aware of the value of eating sunflower seeds I left the house on the farm one day for a walk but had to return after being out only a moment, as the excessive brightness of the snow interfered with my vision. In fact, it made the snow seem a pink color. After being on the sunflower diet for about a month I noticed I could walk in the snow without distress. A little while later my car broke down and I had to walk over a mile on a snowed-up highway in bright sunshine with no trouble at all for the first three-quarters of the way. On the last stretch the eyes smarted a little.

He went on to say that after publishing his first article on sunflower seeds in an early issue of *Organic Gardening* magazine people began to eat the seeds and letters poured in by the hundreds testifying to the benefits. Here are a few representative examples of the correspondence he received:

"Sunflower seeds have done a lot of good for me. I needed reading glasses since I was 45 years old, am 65 now, have eaten the seeds for about two years or more and can read a lot now without glasses."–J.W.E.

"I brought my eyesight back with sunflower seeds, three teaspoonfuls of the kernels a day. Everything was a blur, but now I can read without glasses. Even my hair is getting life and luster back into it."–Mrs. E.M.

"After reading Mr. Rodale's booklet on *Sunflower Seed, the Miracle Food,* and having had severe eye trouble for many years, I decided to try the seeds. I ate a good-sized handful each day and in about two weeks I noticed a definite and almost unbelievable change. The strain, ache, and pain almost completely disappeared and I could work the entire day without being conscious of any trouble. An eye specialist (one of the best in North Carolina) after an examination stated that my eyes had improved and he prescribed weaker lenses."–R.D.B.

"About six weeks ago I read your booklet about sunflower seeds. I was impressed by what eating these seeds had done for others in strengthening their eyes. Mine have always been my most sensitive organs so I immediately got some seeds and thought that I'd try them for one month, as the article said results should be expected in that time. One month—that was good! The very first time I ate sunflower seeds I felt results (let alone a month later)! I knew then and there that sunflower seeds were good for me and something my eyes needed. And the more I have eaten, the better they get. The results are immediate and at the same time lasting."—S.F.C.

"I am 66 years old and have always worn glasses. Have unusually far vision, so objects near were hard to distinguish. As my health improved my glasses did not help, so I used them only for sewing or near work. I have never taken vitamins to any amount. I use about half a cup of sunflower seeds a day. I sprout some and use in salads. As I could not crack shells I pour boiling water over them. Then pour water off. I eat while ironing, walking, while on the bus or while reading or listening to the radio. I can at times thread a needle and sew without the aid of glasses. Often go all day without glasses, which I have not been able to do for many years. I notice I have gained weight. I feel the seeds are really helping me to restore my eyesight."—M.T.

COPING WITH CATARACT

Cataract is a disorder of the eyes in which the lens becomes opaque, like a frosted windowglass. It is not a condition where cells grow abnormally but rather appears to represent cells dying off and turning white in the process.

There are several forms of cataract, but senile cataract is the most common. This type generally afflicts older people but it can and does occur among young persons as well.

How the Strange Name of Cataract Began

The peculiar name for this distressing eye disorder was given by the ancient Greeks. They believed that a cloudy fluid was flowing from the eyes so they called it cataract—a waterfall. Although today we know that the condition is not due to a flow of water, we have still kept the name.

Science Discovers Effective Vitamin Therapy for Cataract

A deficiency of vitamin B-2 (riboflavin) has been shown to cause cataracts in both humans and animals. In experiments conducted by Dr. P. S. Day at Columbia University, rats deprived of vitamin B-2 in their diets all developed cataracts. If sufficient amounts of riboflavin were given early enough, it caused the cataract to disappear and the eyes to become perfectly normal. Cataracts returned when these same test animals were again placed on a riboflavin-deficient diet.

Dr. Sydenstricker of the University of Georgia and University of Georgia Hospital has proved that vitamin B-2 therapy helps humans threatened with cataracts. He first tried vitamin A on 47 patients suffering from various eye ailments—18 of whom had opacities which generally indicate formation of cataract, and six who had fully developed cataracts. Although vitamin A is a nutrient known to be essential for eye health and effective in treating various types of eye disorders it did not produce the desired effects in the 47 patients.

Dr. Sydenstricker then prescribed 15 milligrams of vitamin B-2 daily. This was the only treatment used. Dramatic improvement was noted within 24 hours. In almost every case the burning sensations and other symptoms such as itching, general eye weakness, and faulty vision began to disappear. Those showing no improvement within the first 24 hours were relieved within the next 24 hours. After continued use (nine months) of riboflavin therapy, cataract patients found their cataracts had been reabsorbed and their eyes had become perfectly normal.

In order to prove the effectiveness of the riboflavin therapy, Dr. Sydenstricker placed a few of the cured patients back on a diet deficient in vitamin B-2. Before long, the same eye symptoms returned, and were once again corrected by administration of riboflavin.

Sources of Vitamin B-2

Brewer's yeast is the richest source of riboflavin (one heaping tablespoonful contains approximately 2.175 mg of vitamin B-2). Other excellent sources are sprouted grains, and muscle and organ meats such as liver.

OTHER TREATMENTS FOR CATARACT

A homeopathic tincture made from the herb *Cineraria maritima* is reported to have produced good results in some cases of cataract.

All opacities of the eye, corneal or vitreous, are best treated with *Cineraria maritima.* The homeopathic tincture of *Cineraria* is famous as the most effective means of controlling early forms of cataract. One or two drops in each eye morning and night where there is any sign of trouble is the best safeguard against the development of cataract. Many established early cataracts have been halted and cleared by the prompt and regular use of *Cineraria.*[6]

Other qualified sources also report that the most satisfactory results are attained when the preparation is used in the early stages of cataract. In these cases, clinical experience and observations have shown decided benefits in arresting or even dissolving existing opacities by local applications of this homeopathic herbal remedy.

Advanced Cases of Cataract

A study was conducted by ophthalmologists (medical eye specialists) to obtain more data regarding the effects of *Cineraria maritima* in advanced conditions of cataract. It was used in 40 cases in which the onset of the disease was over four years. This is past the stage where best results are obtainable. Two drops of the liquid were placed in the eyes of each patient morning and night. Results showed that 22.5 percent of the group of 40 patients received beneficial effects. Considering that the condition of cataract in these cases was beyond the early stage, the results are especially impressive.

NATURAL REMEDIES FOR VARIOUS EYE TROUBLES

Glaucoma

"This disease requires careful professional attention with dietary changes and control of fluid intake to reduce the condition. But dosage with very small amounts of homeopathic gelsemium under supervision will produce excellent results."[7]

Some nutritionists have found that glaucoma patients are usually deficient in vitamins A, B, and C, along with calcium and other minerals.

Dr. R. Ulrich forbids his glaucoma patients to drink coffee as he believes there is a connection between coffee and glaucoma.

---

[6] *Acta Phytotherapeutica,* Vol. XII, No. 9.

[7] *Fitness,* July 1964.

Corneal Ulcers

1. *"Hydrastis* [golden seal] tincture or fluid extract applied externally to the cornea in a dilution of two drops in an eye bath will heal a corneal ulcer if used three times daily."[8]
2. In a test among 51 patients suffering from deep corneal ulcers it was found that large doses (1500 mg.) of vitamin C daily resulted in impressive and quick healing.

Vitamin C is not stored in the body so you must get it every day from herbs or foods containing vitamin C, or you may use vitamin C tablets. Rose hips and acerola berries are rich natural sources of this important vitamin.

Spots Before the Eyes

"In many cases of 'floaters' or 'spots before the eyes' the trouble is due to congested liver and should be treated with diet and medicines which normalize the function of the liver."[9]

Reported Remedies for Bags Under the Eyes

Unattractive bags under the eyes are sometimes caused by water retention. However the most common cause is sleep loss, so along with getting enough sleep you may try either of the following remedies. (The selected remedy should be used daily until results have been achieved.)

1. Steep two papaya tea bags (which can be bought in health food stores) in a cup of boiling water. Lie down in a relaxed, comfortable position and apply the tea bags warm, not hot, to the area under the eyes for 15 minutes.
2. Grated cucumber may be applied instead of the papaya tea bags. It imparts a sense of freshness, and excellent results have been reported with its use.
3. Peel and grate a small potato and apply. Allow to remain for 15 minutes.

Note: The last two remedies have also been found effective in helping to eliminate dark circles under the eyes when the condition is due to lack of sleep.

---

[8] *Acta Phytotherapeutica,* Vol. XII, No. 9.
[9] Ibid.

Bloodshot Eyes

To correct or prevent the condition of bloodshot eyes, nutritionists suggest the B vitamin foods with particular attention to vitamin B-2–brewer's yeast, sprouted grains, etc.

Granulated Eyelids

Evidence has shown that itching or granulation of the eyelids, or irritation of the whites of the eyes, are indications of riboflavin deficiency. A person lacking in this vitamin often wipes or rubs his eyes.

Tired Eyes

1. Don't throw away your used ordinary tea bags. Instead hang them up and dry carefully. When your eyes feel tired, reheat the tea bags with hot water, and when comfortably warm place them over the closed eyelids. Allow to remain on for three to five minutes. Rinse with clear cool water. This simple treatment is very refreshing for tired eyes.
2. Here is another suggestion: Place fresh slices of cucumber over the closed eyelids.
3. Pads soaked with diluted witch hazel or rosemary tea will cool and refresh tired eyes.

Alleviating Sties of the Eyes

Castor oil applied externally is a favorite folk remedy for clearing up sties. One woman wrote: "With me a sty only lasts a few days when anointed with castor oil. A friend of mine had a bad sty. I advised her to use the oil. She did so. She was amazed at its disappearance within two or three days. She passed on the information to another woman whose eyes were troubled in this way, and that lady too was surprised at an almost immediate response. How long will it be before we return to the older and more reliable medicines of proven worth?"

Drs. Wood and Ruddock recommend drinking a tea made from the seeds or roots of burdock as a highly effective remedy for sties. "A pint of the infusion may be drunk in the course of 24 hours." As a preventive method for those troubled by recurring sties, "Make a strong tea of burdock seeds or ground centaury plant and take a tablespoonful three or four times a day."

Here is another simple remedy suggested by the two physicians: "On the first appearance of the sty put two teaspoonfuls of black tea in a small sack, moisten with hot water, bind it on the eyelid while warm, and retain it there overnight. If applied in time, one application is sufficient to remove the sty. Sometimes the second or third application may be necessary. If the tea is moistened with warm water two or three times during the night, it will have better effect."

CHAPTER SUMMARY

1. A number of troublesome eye conditions can be relieved and often overcome with the use of herbs.
2. Teas, compresses, eye baths, eye lotions, and homeopathic preparations are various ways in which the herbs are employed.
3. Eyebright herb has an ancient and world-wide reputation as a specific remedy for some forms of eye distress.
4. Certain vitamins and minerals contained in certain herbs are necessary for protecting and maintaining eye health.
5. Sunflower seeds, brewer's yeast, parsley, and other specific herbs and natural foods are rich nutritional factors that contribute to desirable eye health.

4

How Herbs Can Help
Build Your Blood for
a More Youthful Vitality

Vibrant health, youthful vigor and vitality start with a clean, pure bloodstream. The blood goes everywhere; it feeds and nourishes all parts of the body, and also acts as a barrier against disease. A revitalized, reactivated bloodstream can help you attain robust health reflected by youthful appearance, whereas a disordered condition of the blood can result in illness and premature aging. A prominent professor of nutrition once said: "If I had been sick 200 years ago, I would have been better off in the hands of a medicine man of the American Indians than I would have been in those of a European physician. The Indian would have given me mental therapy, food and herb remedies. The European physician would have drained away my blood!" ("Bleeding" a patient of his blood was a common therapy years ago.)

HERBS AND NATURAL FOODS FOR COPING WITH
IRON-POOR BLOOD

An important step in building or regaining youthful energy and stamina is to bring your body's stores of iron up to par. Iron is absolutely essential for the formation of rich red blood. A deficiency of this precious mineral can cause headaches, pallor of the face and lips, depression, crying spells, listlessness, weakness, exhaustion, and other debilitating problems.

Women require more iron than men do, partly because they have fewer red blood cells to begin with, but mainly because of the demands that menstruation and pregnancy make upon the blood and its constituents. Over 80 percent of the iron in the human body is found in the red blood cells, therefore loss of blood through menstruation means loss of iron. Iron loss in menstruating women is estimated to be about 30 milligrams every month.

The recommended daily dietary allowance of iron for all females from 10 to 55 years of age is 18 milligrams. Yet surveys over the past years have consistently shown that the fair sex consumes an average of only about 10 or 11 milligrams of iron per day. As a result, many women suffer from borderline anemia and are unable to function at their best.

Copper Also Needed

In the *Journal of Biological Chemistry,* an article on "The Action of Copper in Iron Metabolism" tells us that although the body can assimilate iron without copper, it cannot utilize iron for regeneration of the hemoglobin unless copper is included in the diet. The hemoglobin is the red pigment of blood that carries oxygen. When your brain isn't getting enough oxygen you can't think clearly, or remember names or dates. Furthermore, you can't really seem to play a good game of bowling or enjoy a swim or other recreational activities because you're too soon breathless and exhausted.

Chemical Iron Compounds

In conditions of iron deficiency, physicians frequently prescribe ferrous sulfate or ferrous gluconate. Many people who have used a ferrous compound have found that it tends to constipate, or that it irritates the stomach or bowels. According to *Merck Index* even an average dose of either of the ferrous compounds can cause gastrointestinal irritation; however, the ferrous gluconate causes less discomfort than the sulfate.

Organic Iron from Plants

Organic iron rarely disagrees with the human system and can be obtained from certain herbs and unrefined foods for those who suspect they may be suffering from borderline anemia or who are wise enough to want to protect themselves against this debilitating condition. For example, distributed over a wide area of the country is a remarkable plant called yellow dock *(Rumex crispus)* whose root is a veritable storehouse of organic iron, combined with copper. Along with these valuable constituents, yellow dock root also contains mild laxative properties. An infusion prepared from the root of this gentle herb will not irritate, bind, or constipate.

The Secret of Preparing Yellow Dock Tea for Maximum Benefits

Although hard plant substances such as roots or barks are generally boiled for a certain length of time in order to extract their properties, yellow dock root is an exception and *must never be boiled* as boiling destroys its valuable constituents. Yellow dock tea is simply made by adding from one to one and a half teaspoonfuls of the cut root to a cup of piping hot water. The tea is covered with a saucer and allowed to stand for 20 minutes. It is then strained, reheated, and taken in sips—one cup three times a day. The tea may be flavored with lemon or honey.

Other Natural Sources of Iron

Another remarkably rich source of natural iron with strong hemoglobin regeneration power is wheat germ. It also supplies copper, manganese, and the B vitamins, all of which are important to iron utilization.

Here is a table listing some of the many plant foods high in natural organic iron:

Food	Amount	Milligrams of Iron
Almonds	1/2 cup	3.3
Apricots, dried, uncooked	1/2 cup	4.1
Beans, baked	1 cup	4.7
Beans, kidney, canned	1 cup	4.9
Beet greens, steamed	1/2 cup	1.4
Brussel sprouts, steamed	1 cup	1.7

Dandelion greens, steamed	1 cup	5.5
Dates	1 cup	5.7
Lentils	1 cup	4.1
Molasses, blackstrap	1 tablespoon	2.3
Mustard greens, steamed	1 cup	4.1
Parsley, raw, chopped	2 tablespoons	.4
Prune juice	1 cup	9.8
Radishes	5 large	1.0
Raisins	1/2 cup	2.8
Soybeans	1 cup	5.4
Soy flour, full fat	1 cup	8.8
Tomato juice	1/2 cup	1.1
Turnip greens, steamed	1 cup	3.5
Wheat germ	1 cup	5.5
Whole wheat flour	1 cup	3.0
Yeast, brewer's	1/4 cup	5.0

NATURE'S BLOOD CLEANSERS

Another function the Creator has allotted to the bloodstream is that of providing the elements needed to neutralize and carry away toxins and impurities caused by metabolism, cell disintegration, etc. When toxins are allowed to accumulate in the bloodstream any number of diseases can result. Experiments by Carrel and Woodruff showed that a regular "washing out" of waste products in cell cultures helped prolong the life of the cells indefinitely.

Fresh fruit and fruit juices are excellent blood cleansers, whereas raw vegetables and vegetable juices are considered builders and regenerators. Dr. Bircher-Benner of Zurich, Switzerland, who uses mostly raw juices and raw foods in his health sanitarium, said: "Absorption and organization of sunlight, the essence of life, takes place almost exclusively within the plants. The organs of the plants are therefore a kind of biological accumulation of light. They are the basis of what we call *food*, whence animal and human bodies derive their substance and energy. Nutritional energy may thus be termed organized light energy."

One-Day Fast with Fruit Juices

Eating nothing but fresh fruit or drinking only fresh fruit juices one day a week or every two weeks or once a month is a very old practice of blood purification which has never lost its popularity. According to news reports, movie star Mae West, who never ceases to amaze people by her youthful appearance, at age 79, said: "You know the body continually renews itself, and with proper food and proper internal cleansing of the system, age won't set in as fast as it would otherwise. Once a week I take six oranges, three grapefruit and two lemons, squeeze the juice out, add the same amount of distilled water, and have nothing but that for nourishment the whole day. It gives my insides a chance to relax and take it easy and get cleaned out."

HERBAL BLOOD CLEANSERS

The early herb doctors searched for herbs that would help do the job of eliminating impurities from the blood. Plants used for this purpose were, and still are, called "blood purifiers" in the broad sense of the term. In modern herbalism they are often employed as a treatment for skin diseases which arise from a disordered condition of the blood.

Fragrant Spicy Sassafras

Sassafras, for example, has long been known and used as a "spring tonic" for clearing the blood and toning up the system generally. Du Pratz called it the "great tree" of medicine. William Byrd claimed that the berries, fruit, and rind were effective for treating a variety of illnesses, and further that the flowers mixed in salads and eaten in the spring were excellent blood cleansers.

In 1830, Rafinesque wrote a complete description of this spicy American tree and its medicinal employment, stating among other things that the "Indians use a strong decoction to purge and clear the body in the spring, we use instead the tea or blossoms for a venal purification of the blood." John Lighthall suggested that people make a tea of sassafras and "drink it either warm or cold at meals instead of store tea or coffee, and during the day instead of water when you have bad blood."

Sassafras Still Popular

Today, the reputation of sassafras as a home-remedy spring tonic and blood purifier has remained unchanged, and its medicinal value in some areas has been scientifically acknowledged. The root-bark prepared in the form of the usual decoction offers a fragrant, refreshing, and healthful beverage. "Sassafras bars" are built near popular health resorts, where the tea is served either cold or piping hot.

Constituents in Sassafras

The bark of sassafras root contains a volatile oil, resin, wax, camphor, fatty matter, albumen, starch, gum, lignin, tannic acid, salts, and a decomposition product of tannic acid known as *sassafrid.* It has been found to possess general antiseptic power in various instances.

A Remedy for Skin Disorders

According to a leading journal of organic medicine, sassafras combined in the following manner with other appropriate herbs provides a valuable remedy for varied skin disorders, such as eczema:

> Red clover flowers, 2 oz.; burdock root, 1 oz.; blue flag root, 1 oz.; sassafras bark, ½ oz.
> Method: Place one-quarter of the mixture in one pint of cold water, bring to a boil, simmer for 20 minutes, strain when cold.
> Dose: One wineglassful three times daily, until improvement is apparent.

Burdock—Another Favorite Herb Blood Cleanser

Burdock *(Arctium lappa)* is another plant which has long enjoyed a reputation as a blood cleanser. An early edition of the *U. S. Dispensatory* mentions its value in skin disorders with the following instructions: "To prove effectual its administration must be long continued; a pint may be given daily of the decoction made by boiling two ounces of the root in three pints of water down to two pints."

William Smith, N.D., F.N.I.M.H., a practicing medical herbalist of modern times, calls burdock "one of the finest blood purifiers" and advises that "both root and seeds should be prepared as a decoction with one ounce to one and a half pints of water which is simmered down to one pint and taken in wineglassful doses three or four times daily. It may be combined, if required, with yellow dock and sarsaparilla."

Scientific analyses reveal that burdock contains vitamin C, iron, niacin, inulin, mucilage, sugar, a little resin, tannic acid, fixed and volatile oils, and a bitter crystalline glucoside. In Europe the root is used in herbal blood purifying mixtures and pills.

Included among the many other herbs regarded as blood cleansers we find red clover, nettle, echinacea, parsley, poke root, yellow dock, sarsaparilla, watercress, oregon grape root, and violet.

CONSTIPATION AND ASSOCIATED AUTOINTOXICATION

Constipation, called "the great American tragedy," is perhaps the most common health problem in our country. Kellog was of the opinion that this problem and associated autointoxication are the causes of most human ailments. Autointoxication, resulting from absorption into the blood stream of toxic fecal waste products, is one of the chief causes of old age, according to Professor Metchnikoff, a Russian physiologist. He maintained that prevention of such intoxication would help preserve youth and prolong life beyond the so-called normal span.

Regular daily evacuations of the bowels, then, is another important step in maintaining or rebuilding a clean pure bloodstream that can keep you feeling youthful and healthy. However, it is generally agreed by almost everyone that drugs and laxatives do more harm than good in coping with the problem of constipation. So let us consider some of the experiences of others in using natural methods for dealing with sluggish bowels.

PERSONAL EXPERIENCES OF THOSE WHO
OVERCAME CONSTIPATION[1]

Less Milk—More Fruit

"My experience with laxatives ended abruptly four years ago after a five-day period of hospitalization with asthma. Before entering the hospital I practically never had a bowel movement except after drinking sauerkraut juice. Upon my return home, I decided on a very simple diet change: less bread and milk, more fruits, vegetables and meats. The change was designed to help my chronic asthmatic condition.

"Although it has not been entirely successful in this respect it did immediately correct constipation. Not once in the last four years have I ever taken any kind of laxative and not once during this time have I been constipated."—D.E.J.

Brewer's Yeast

"I would like to tell you of my husband's experiences with brewer's yeast tablets. My husband was a CVA patient in a medical hospital for six weeks, during which time he never had a normal or natural evacuation. It was a steady round of physics, enemas, and impactions. When he came home I immediately started him on yeast tablets and within a week he was having natural and comfortable evacuations and has continued to do so for six months."—Mrs. J.A.G.

Crown to Sunflower Seeds

"I want to say that sunflower seeds wear the crown when it comes to regularity. They act as a laxative and also provide the body with much good nutrition, so they can't help but improve general health. I buy sunflower seeds in bulk and distribute them at cost to my friends. One friend was constipated for years. Sunflower seeds were the answer for him."—F.E.B.

Combination Vital

"I was cured of constipation by taking a heaping teaspoon of raw wheat germ and brewer's yeast powder with each meal. I was

---

[1]All references *Prevention*, March 1966.

out of wheat germ for a while and just took the brewer's yeast and got constipated again."—Mrs. G.W.I.

Raw Fruit

"I used to be constipated all the time for years, getting relief only from enemas. Now, after eating raw fruit and taking many food supplements, I have two or three bowel movements a day."—Mrs. T.H.

Blackstrap Molasses

"My husband was bothered with constipation for years and had to rely on pills for several years until a friend told him to take a tablespoon of crude blackstrap unsulphured molasses in the morning and at night when retiring. It has done the job and he doesn't need the pills now."—Mrs. G.A.

Tomatoes, Not Juice

"I eat two or three tomatoes before breakfast, and I find this helps me to stay regular because it is 'life food' and not juice out of a can."—D.J.T.

No Bread, No Trouble

"Having experienced a lifetime's annoyance with constipation, it finally came to a point this year when there would be complete stoppage at times. I swore off on all drug laxatives over 40 years ago as I found nothing that would eliminate the cause of the trouble.

"Two months ago I cut out bread completely and supplemented it with sunflower and pumpkin seeds and the results are that there have been regular movements ever since."—T.G.W.

COPING WITH CHOLESTEROL

Among all degenerative changes blamed for premature aging, short life-span, and death, none has received more attention than atherosclerosis, commonly called "hardening of the arteries."

Cholesterol is a major ingredient of plaque, a build-up of fatty particles that frequently become deposited within the arteries. When the arteries become clogged, blood circulation to all parts of the body is reduced, especially to the brain. This shortage of blood to the brain can cause mental confusion, forgetfulness, and high blood pressure. A young person can also develop these same conditions if his arteries are clogged, thus experiencing premature aging.

Deposits of fatty particles also cause the heart to work harder in order to pump the blood through the clogged passageways. Here is where many heart and coronary troubles begin, if the heart is forced to undertake more work than it is able to do.

The Magic of Lecithin in Soybeans

Scientific studies are proving that none of these conditions need develop in anyone, young or old. Lecithin, a constituent of soybeans, has the ability to break up fatty substances such as cholesterol, thereby discouraging the formation of plaques within the artery walls.

In a study by Dr. Robert Hodges of the University of Iowa, a group of healthy volunteers were fed a soybean meat substitute. Later, the doctor found that their levels of cholesterol had been reduced from an average of approximately 300 milligrams per cubic centimeter of serum to 200 and less. Dr. Hodges stated that the average cholesterol level in most Americans is about 240 and higher.

According to a report cited in an issue of *Geriatrics*,[2] two tablespoonfuls (36 grams) of lecithin given every day to high cholesterol patients with hardening of the arteries brought a 41 percent drop in cholesterol levels in 13 out of 15 patients.

The staff of the *British Medical Journal*[3] recommends soybean oil for treating an excess of cholesterol in the blood. The oil may also help in preventing blood clots and heart attacks.

The Go-Power in Soybeans

Along with their rich content of unsaturated fat, of which the most important is lecithin, soybeans provide an abundance of

[2]January 1958.
[3]October 16, 1965.

protein, vital to tissue growth and repair. Protein is also a valuable factor in maintaining the health of the blood and arteries. In a study by Dr. D. Davis of West Wales General Hospital, it was revealed that patients with coronary artery disease showed a deficiency of blood serum proteins necessary for antibody activity. Dr. Davis suggested that without sufficient protein, changes in metabolic patterns of the blood might prepare the stage for atherosclerosis.

Soybeans are also rich in vitamins A, E, K, and some of the B factors. Potassium, a mineral required to maintain fluid balance in the tissues, is also plentiful in soybeans. Along with these valuable nutrients the beans contain good quantities of iron, phosphorus, calcium and amino acids. The minerals present in soybeans play an important role in preventing cardiovascular disorders. According to scientific studies, a shortage of these elements in the body appears to go hand in hand with atherosclerosis.

Vitamin C, so abundant in soybean sprouts, has also been found helpful in reducing cholesterol build-up in the liver, brain, and heart.

How Soybeans May Be Used in Your Diet

There are many ways to utilize soybeans in your diet. Soybean flakes or grits make excellent breakfast foods; you can use soy sauce for flavoring your meat; soybeans can be steamed, baked, mixed with tomato sauce or corn, or you can roast the kernels; soybean milk makes a healthful beverage; soy flour can replace white flour; soybean oil may be used in cooking or in salads; lecithin soy powders are also available as supplements to help control cholesterol levels.

OTHER STUDIES ON CHOLESTEROL-REDUCING PROGRAMS

In his book, *The Low-Fat Way to Health and Longer Life,*[4] Dr. Lester M. Morrison writes: "I am going to tell you about one of the most important nutritional supplements developed in the last 50 years. Make a careful note of it and of how it is to be used, as described in these pages. The least it can do for you is to improve

[4]Englewood Cliffs, N.J.: Prentice-Hall, Inc., 1958.

your health and give you added vitality. And it may even help save your life.

"The substance is Lecithin—a bland, water-soluble, granular powder made from de-fatted soya beans."

After many years of careful analyses and evaluation of the results, Dr. Morrison says that he is "certain that Lecithin is one of our most powerful weapons against disease. It is an especially valuable bulwark against development of 'hardening of the arteries' and all the complications of heart, brain, and kidney that follow." He also feels that soya oil is "the most healthful of all food oils."

In studying the effects of food and nutritional supplement programs recommended to a large number of patients, Dr. Morrison reports that they brought about a lessening of nervousness, constipation and fatigue, and a decrease in the number of infections and colds that patients usually had. "Also of greatest importance was the fact that they were found to be instrumental in lowering the cholesterol content of the blood and in reducing the amount of harmful blood fats."

Five-Step Program

Dr. Morrison asked his patients to employ the following five-step program:

1. Include daily as a food supplement at breakfast two to four tablespoonfuls of Lecithin extracted from soya beans.
2. Add to your diet each day B Complex vitamins in the most potent form. Avoid the cheaper preparations which provide only small and ineffectual quantities of the vitamins, and have little or no effect on the body. Your doctor or druggist can advise you which brands provide potent quantities of the vitamins.
3. Also add to your daily diet at least 25,000 units of vitamin A, and 150 mg. of vitamin C.[5]
4. Take two tablespoonfuls of soya bean oil, corn oil or safflower oil daily to provide the essential fatty acids necessary to proper nutrition. The oil may be used as a

---

[5]Many nutritionalists feel that 500 to 1000 mg. of vitamin C is now needed.

salad dressing, taken with tomato or fruit juice, or used in any way you prefer.

5. Include in your diet two to four tablespoonfuls of whole wheat germ each day. This may be eaten as a breakfast cereal with fruit, or sprinkled on your salad.

Other Remarkable Benefits Provided by Lecithin

Referring again to the value of lecithin, Dr. Morrison says, "In some instances, the cosmetic effect of Lecithin did as much for the patients' mental outlook as it did for their physical well-being.

"For example, Mrs. U., a housewife of 45, had always been ashamed of the flat plaques of yellowish hue that appeared on her skin owing to fatty deposits. Soon after she began adding Lecithin to her diet, as prescribed, the patches began to disappear. Eventually they vanished altogether. Mrs. U. was more delighted with what she saw happening in the mirror than with the idea that the same thing might be going on with the fatty deposits inside her arteries."

Dr. Morrison also tells us, "Lecithin has other remarkable therapeutic qualities as well. One that we are just beginning to explore is its ability to increase the gamma globulin content of the blood proteins. These gamma globulins are known to be associated with nature's protective force against the attacks of various infections in the body.

"In the bloodstream of patients who used Lecithin as recommended, we found evidence of increased immunity against virus infections. This is of special interest, since scientists have reported finding this Lecithin-induced immunity against pneumonia."

Three-Way Combination

Years of research have convinced Dr. Morrison and his co-workers of the value of the following ideal nutritional combination on patients suffering from high blood pressure, strokes, and other ailments resulting from hardening of the arteries: "(a) Low-fat, high protein diet; (b) large amounts of vitamin B complex, together with lipotropic (fat-preventing) agents such as choline, betaine, and inosital (all members of the vitamin B complex); and (c) nutritional supplements such as liver extract, lecithin, and brewer's yeast."

Swedish Report

Dr. Morrison calls attention to a Swedish report in which remarkable improvements in older people were brought about with the use of the low-fat, low-cholesterol diet he had originally recommended, consisting of only 25 grams of fat each day. The program was prescribed by Drs. G. Lindquist and B. Isaksson at the University of Gothenburg Hospital for 19 hospital patients, men and women ranging from 50 to 87 years of age. In addition to the low-fat, low-cholesterol diet, some were also given a supply of multiple vitamins daily. Dr. Morrison says, "All patients, with one exception, had suffered from a stroke or cerebral thrombosis as a result of hardening of the brain arteries." As a result of their strokes the patients had experienced some paralysis or disability of the legs, hands, or muscles of the arm. They also showed symptoms of mental depression, weakness, listlessness, nervousness, and despair.

Dr. Morrison points out that patients of this type "whose number is tragically legion, are generally regarded by most physicians as hopeless and are simply to be kept alive as long as possible." He adds that, "Many doctors still view these pathetic people as the inevitable result of old age, the results of wear-and-tear of the arteries—the hardening of the arteries in the brain."

The patients in the Swedish report were placed on the low-fat nutrition program for three months. At the end of that time most of them showed amazing improvement mentally, emotionally, and physically. The ability for endurance and concentration was markedly increased. This was evident from the way the patients applied themselves to the physical exercises which were part of the treatment for weak muscles and paralysis. Dr. Morrison says that "some of the patients made such extraordinary mental and physical progress that they were sufficiently well to be discharged from the hospital."

Case Histories

He then discusses many case histories of elderly patients under his own care. One was an 83-year-old woman who was brought to his office in a wheel chair. The patient was almost blind, partly deaf, and too feeble to walk or to feed herself. Two months of the following treatment was prescribed: "Large amounts of natural and synthetic vitamins, plus nutritional supplements, such as lecithin, soya oil and liver extract were given in addition to the low-fat, high-protein diet. Under our very eyes a nutritional miracle then took place. Mrs. A. walked in to see me, under her own power. She was able to see, even though not as clearly as at one time. Because her hearing had returned, we were able to carry on a conversation. And I found—marvelous to behold!—that she still had a sense of humor. She was able to poke fun at herself and spoke of my 'robbing the grave.' "

Another Remarkable Case

"Or take the case of Miss R., a 65-year-old maiden lady who had a stroke or cerebral thrombosis, the result of atherosclerosis. Her vision was failing and she was partly paralyzed, desperate, and depressed. Except for one friend, she was all alone in the world."

Dr. Morrison says that after several months of using the low-fat nutritional program as described in his book, "Miss R. recovered much of her muscular power, her partial paralysis gradually disappeared, and she became a radiant picture of cheerfulness and optimism. Her vision had greatly improved, and when last seen in my office she asked me brightly, 'Doctor, could I go swimming?' I replied, 'Indeed yes, but—no diving!' "

CHAPTER SUMMARY

1. A clean well-nourished blood stream flowing through heart and brain, and supplying every organ, tissue and gland with the necessary nutrients through herbals, promotes the basis of good health.

2. Iron is essential for the formation of rich, red blood. A deficiency of this mineral can cause a number of debilitating health problems. Certain herbals supply organic sources of iron.
3. Women require more iron than men do, mainly because of the demands that menstruation and pregnancy make upon the blood and its constituents.
4. Organic iron rarely disagrees with the human system, and can be obtained from certain herbs and natural foods.
5. When impurities are allowed to accumulate and pollute the bloodstream, illness and symptoms of premature aging can result.
6. Certain herbs are natural and efficient blood cleansers.
7. Herbs can be used in coping with hardening of the arteries.

5

Selected Herbs to Help Grow and Promote a Beautiful Head of Hair

Hair has always been regarded as a woman's crowning glory and a man's symbol of masculine vigor and strength. Although hair is not essential to life, it is of sufficient cosmetic concern to provoke anxiety in anyone when it starts thinning, falling, or disappearing.

To a woman, the sight of a brush covered with lost hairs can cause hysteria. According to Dr. Howard T. Behrman, dermatologist of New York Medical College: "All women tend to become hysterical, and some psychotic, at the thought of impending baldness." And worry caused by hair loss only makes matters worse, as it aggravates the condition of hair loss.

Female Baldness

The type of baldness prevalent among females never becomes the horseshoe hairline that afflicts so many men. A woman's problem is a thinning out of the hair that gets progressively worse, then eventually stops. The scalp can be seen through the hair but it is not swept clean. In some cases, however, the hair may fall out in patches, leaving a small bald spot here and there, but these are exceptions rather than the general rule.

In brief, although the problem may be psychologically catastrophic, baldness among women is not as severe as the type of hair loss that plagues men. Another point on the plus side for the ladies is that female baldness is easier to remedy.

Male Baldness Pattern

Among men who have a baldness problem, especially the young male, the loss is most disturbing in the early stages. Generally, a man's first reaction to the onset of a receding hairline is one of shock and a feeling of disfigurement. He also associates hair loss with weakness, an idea that goes far back in time, the classical example being that of Samson, who lost his great strength after Delilah clipped his manly locks. He feels, too, that his image as a sex symbol is on the way to being sharply curtailed. With the passage of time the chain of anxieties set up by hair loss becomes progressively deeper, and severe psychological damage may also result.

To put it simply, hair-fall makes life miserable for some 12 million American men who have a barren scalp where a flowing mane once used to be. And the misery of this sizable minority is compounded by frustration and disappointment after spending millions of dollars for hair restoratives that don't grow a single hair.

Male pattern baldness is an age-old problem, and the aim of developing an effective anti-balding remedy ranks as one of the most elusive goals known to man. Treatments have ranged from a mixture of animal fats (a prescription recorded on the Ebers papyrus sheets over 5000 years ago) to present techniques featuring electric lamps, ultra-sonics, hair lotions, massage and diathermy. But the repeated pattern of these methods has been one of mere promises, and inevitable failure.

Some Facts About Hair

If you are blond you have approximately 140,000 hairs on your head; somewhat less—about 110,000—if you are brunette; and around 90,000 if you have red hair. The pigment which gives your hair its color is situated in the central layer of the hair called the cortex. As hair grows, the old hair moves up inside the follicle, depositing a column of cells behind it which will form new hair. In normal conditions the rate of replacement keeps pace with the rate of loss, but if the hair which falls out does not deposit the vital growing nucleus there will be no new growth to replace it. Baldness is the inevitable result of hair loss exceeding hair growth.

The hair follicle itself is surrounded by sebaceous glands and sweat glands. An oily substance called sebum, which is secreted by the sebaceous glands, in excessive amounts results in an oily scalp or hair.

The scaling off of old skin is a natural process which takes place in all areas of the body but is more apparent on the scalp where it collects. Dandruff is the result of an unhealthy scalp condition in which too much of the skin is scaling off. Seborrhea is a much more serious condition in which the secretion of the sebaceous gland is excessive and oily scales of dandruff result.

Your hair, like your fingernails, is basically protein.

BALDNESS AMONG WOMEN

Women's Crowning Glory in Decline

For years the number of balding women was minimal and the trend remained unchanged. Then suddenly around the mid-1950's the number of women suffering from hair loss doubled, then tripled, and before long that number doubled again. By the time 1962 rolled around, the number of balding women had increased by 122%. (Today, reports indicate that one out of every three women has a hair loss problem!)

A similar increase was reported world wide—from France, Italy, Russia, Britain, and other countries.

Doctors dug deeply into their medical literature searching for clues and found a multitude of possible answers: chemical additives in commercial shampoos and hair preparations, drugs, air pollution, unbalanced nutritional intake from fad diets, tight hair styles, emotional stress. All these factors are known to have damaging effects on the hair, and in this last generation there has been increased contact with these potential causes.

Women Largely to Blame for Their Own "Dis-Tresses"

Reports by experts state that an appalling number of women are responsible for their own hair loss, traceable to prolonged use or misuse of harsh chemical hair preparations, tight binding hair styles, or other questionable cosmetic practices. For example, in

25 cases of baldness among young girls in which the ponytail hair style was used it was found that hair loss began with signs of redness and scaling around the tightened hair follicles. After several months the pulled areas were devoid of hairs and had a "plucked" look. "Teasing" is another bad practice which has been shown to be a particularly brutal technique of combing which can seriously damage the hair if done every day.

According to a leading medical association, permanent wave solutions can act as a depilatory (hair remover), if allowed to remain on the hair too long.

In London several researchers analyzed 95 cases of baldness in women and found that nearly half were caused by harsh hair cosmetics. Dr. S. Alexander reported that 21 of the victims were bald due to the use of hair straighteners; three had suffered hair damage from bleaching and permanent wave solutions; 15 had lost their hair because of the tight hair rollers they had used. In most of these women their crowning glory returned after they quit using whatever caused the baldness.

Dangers Compounded

Along with the potentially damaging effects on the hair, some chemical hair preparations can harm the body. For almost every preparation some person or persons experience an adverse reaction. Do you want to gamble on whether or not you're one of them? Here are a few examples:

Derivatives of coal tar dyes employed in the composition of many shades to change the color of the hair are dangerous. One in particular, phenylenediamine, can be a source of real trouble as it has a high sensitizing potential (an agent which may not cause a noticeable inflamed condition when first applied, but gradually stimulates the production of an allergic reaction). Dr. James W. Burks, writing in "Dermatitis Due to Cosmetics,"[1] calls the reaction to this dye "explosive." It causes tightening of the scalp which is followed by pain, tenderness, and later an oozing, acute inflammation.

---

[1]*Journal of the Southern Medical Association*, Vol. 55, No. 10, October 1962.

Prolonged use of metallic dyes such as silver and lead, sometimes called hair restorers, can have disastrous effects. The silver and lead are slowly absorbed by the body and accumulate in the system. Some of the symptoms of lead poisoning are defective vision, cramps, convulsions, and paralysis. Other hair tonics may contain such poisons as formaldehyde and arsenic, and a dozen irritants such as salicylic acid.

The lacquers, solvents, and other chemicals in hair sprays can cause skin rashes which may spread to other areas of the body. In an article, "Allergies to Cosmetics,"[2] Dr. S.J. Taub says: "Respiratory symptoms such as sneezing, watery eyes, and coughing may also result from their use."

In the *Lancet,* a British medical journal, B.G. Edelston, M.D., reports that inhalation of the synthetic resins of hair sprays is not metabolized in the body and is sometimes found lodged not only in the lungs but also in the liver, spleen, and other organs. These resins cause irritation or inflammation and have been shown to produce lesions on the liver and lungs.

Metallic sprays such as those used for coloring the hair contain finely ground metals such as bronze, copper, silver, and others.

Other Factors Which May Cause Hair Loss

Some of the other factors which can be responsible for hair loss include faulty nutrition which causes the hair papillae to wither and die; severe dandruff; poor circulation to the scalp; certain drugs.

What Can a Woman Do?

Here are some basic rules for preserving your hair and keeping it healthy, and to restore the original crop if it has been thinning out:

1. Quit using harsh chemical hair preparations. Switch to harmless herbal solutions. These are excellent promoters of scalp and hair health, and can easily be prepared right in your own home.

---

[2]*The Eye, Ear, Nose and Throat Monthly,* Vol. 44, August 1965.

2. Avoid tight hair styles, too-tight hair curlers, and rubber bands.
3. Avoid the "teasing" technique of combing the hair.
4. Massage the scalp and brush the hair every day.
5. Never use a nylon brush as it will damage already fine and brittle hair to the breaking point. Some dentists claim that nylon tooth brushes are too hard on the gums and teeth, so imagine what a nylon brush does to your hair! Use a soft, natural bristle brush.
6. Keep the hair and scalp clean by washing with natural herbal shampoos.
7. Steer clear of fad diets that can cause nutritional unbalance. Avoid appetite-depressing drugs.
8. Follow a good nutritional program fortified with plenty of herbs, herbal products, and other vital foods that supply all the nutrients required for a good healthy crop of hair.

Details and instructions for the herbal hair preparations, correct diet, massage and brushing techniques are given further on in this chapter.

BALDNESS AMONG MEN

Why Men Are Losing Their Tops

Any number of things can cause temporary or permanent baldness in the male. For example, scalp infection; physical illnesses of various kinds; chemical hair preparations; drugs; severe dandruff or seborrhea; poor circulation; improper diet. But 90 percent of the cases of hairless scalps are due to what doctors call male pattern baldness. In this condition the hair usually starts receding at the temples; then the hair at the crown begins retreating back and further down the sides, leaving the typical bald spot on top. In severe cases the hapless victim is left with only a fringe of hair circling his head.

A Breakthrough

The generally accepted theories on the cause of male pattern baldness are these: aging; inherited genetic patterns; the male sex hormones. But until recently, science did not know exactly why any of these things produce a barren scalp. Now a Swedish scientist, Dr. Lars Engstrand of Karolinska Institute in Stockholm, has apparently found the answer.

How Male Pattern Baldness Occurs

Dr. Engstrand explains that the tissue-thin membrane which is located on the crown area of the scalp in both men and women is soft and elastic during youth, and in women it remains so throughout life. But with men, the male hormone which produces secondary sex characteristics, voice change, beard growth and body hair, causes the paper-thin membrane of the scalp to thicken. This cuts off the blood supply to the tiny capillaries which are located above the tendinous membrane and which feed the hair follicles with nutrients essential for hair growth. As the thickening process continues over the years, hair growth gradually diminishes until the starving hair follicles eventually atrophy, and the result is baldness.

Dr. Engstrand also points out that aging, hereditary influences, and prolonged mental or emotional stress are other factors which can be involved to some extent in the tendency for developing a thickened membrane. (Modern nutritionalists would add multiple nutritional deficiencies to this list.)

The Swedish scientist has proved his theory of impaired blood supply to the hair roots by performing over 1,000 successful scalp operations which relieved the pressure and resulted in more vigorous hair growth, even on completely bald areas.

What a Man Can Do About It

Aside from surgical treatments, the mainstream of present scientific knowledge holds that male pattern baldness is irreversible; hair once lost is lost forever. Or is it? Modern nutritionalists, biochemists, and endocrinologists have recently presented impressive evidence that the health of the scalp, impaired circulation to the hair roots, and the quality of the blood which feeds the hair can be greatly improved by a diet consisting of vital foods.

Mrs. Katherine Pugh, the first person to formulate a program of hair-through-diet, says: "Anyone who still feels nothing can be done for baldness . . . perhaps has not reviewed the latest findings on hair growth and nutrition." In short, certain herbs, and herbal products such as sunflower seeds, chia seeds, brewer's yeast, wheat germ, wheat germ oil, lecithin (a product of the soya bean), and other power-packed natural foods are your hair's best friend, while sugar, salt, and starches do nothing for a bald scalp. This fact is just as true for women as it is for men.

Feeding the Hair from Within

Mrs. Pugh spent years studying biochemistry and researching documented material from government publications, scientific data, medical journals, both here and abroad. As a result she became convinced that working from the inside by building up the general health would be the logical approach to preventing baldness or restoring hair on an already bald pate. She decided to put the method to work. "I had a bald patch," she said, "and had to comb the hair over it. After I went on a diet of health foods the hair grew in again."

Case History

Later she wrote two books on modern nutrition and its relationship to hair growth.[3] In her writings she describes cases where improved diet stopped hair loss and caused hair to grow again even in advanced conditions of baldness. One is that of a middle-aged man, bald for 20 years—his was the typical male pattern shiny pate with just a fringe around the edges.

One day another member of his household put in a supply of unprocessed foods and he started to eat some of it also, with the result that in about two weeks he noticed hair growth. He said nothing about it, but decided to wait and see if anyone else would notice it. About a week later his astonished wife spotted the tiny hairs coming in on her husband's scalp. Needless to say, the man began to work in earnest to help his hair growth along.

---

[3]Katherine Pugh, *Hair Thru Diet* and *Baldness: Is It Necessary?* (Richmond., Va., 1961.)

Before Mrs. Pugh heard of this case and could get a picture made, six weeks had passed; by that time much of the crown in the back had started filling in and the hair sprouting on the top of the head was about one-half inch long.

According to reports, this man had no scalp disease; his medical history did not reveal any illness; he used no hair tonics, gadgets, or any other form of treatment, local or otherwise. His hair-raising success was apparently due solely to a change of diet.

Another Successful Case

Another case involved that of a man past middle age with a history of weak glands, who was completely bald on top except for a few long hairs.

He had tried ointments, heat lamps, massage and other things. Nothing worked.

When he heard the diet theory he began giving up some of the foods he had formerly eaten and substituting those recommended. He started out by eating sunflower seeds, about one cup for breakfast. Then he tried sunflower seed meal (ground at the time of using), along with pumpkin seed meal and other natural foods. In a few months he noticed a few black hairs at the temple, then he started in earnest to see what he could do about growth.

After about 18 months he noticed a tremendous difference. Hair that was once fuzz was long enough to comb, and a new crop of hair was coming in.

After another 18 months a progress report on this case showed that the subject was doing so well in growing hair that he was able to reduce some of his supplements. He no longer needed to take the B-complex tablets and his doses of vegetable and wheat germ oil were reduced to about one teaspoonful a day. He had also cut down on the amount of meat in his diet.

According to Mrs. Pugh, some younger men have accomplished in weeks what this older man with his sluggish glands and many health problems did in years.

THE DIET THAT BROUGHT HAIR-RAISING RESULTS

You might like to know the dietary routine this man followed. (Keep in mind that later he was able to reduce some of the supplements listed here.)

Sample Day

Breakfast

One kelp tablet (derived from the ocean herb *kelp*) before breakfast.
Two eggs (soft, poached, or scrambled).
Slice of protein bread toast, with soya lecithin spread.
Raw wheat germ and sunflower seed meal mixed to make one-half cup.
Raw fruit in season.
Four high potency B-complex tablets.
25,000 units of vitamin A from fish liver oils.
100 units of vitamin E complex.
Two tablets of iron and liver concentrate.
Two multi-vitamin and mineral tablets.

Lunch

Serving of lean meat, fish or fowl.
One or two green vegetables (or one green vegetable and one low-starch
  vegetable).
Green salad, or cottage cheese, raw cabbage with oil, other salads.
Raw fruit in season.
All *vitamins* same as for breakfast, except vitamin A—it is taken only
  once a day.

Dinner

About the same as for lunch, changing the meat and vegetables for
  variety.
All the vitamins same as breakfast and lunch, with the exception of
  vitamin A.

He takes from one to three tablespoons of oil a day—one of
wheat germ oil and one of any of the vegetable oils, such as soya
oil, sunflower seed oil, others.

He takes the various powders either after meals, as part of the
meal, or between meals, any way that he can work them in, taking
them in juices.

He drinks carrot juice whenever possible.

Sometimes he takes two different brands of B-complex at one
time; in that way he is sure of getting all the B vitamins plus what
he gets in the powders.

Proper Diet Does It

One woman suffered severe hair loss directly following a surgical operation and the loss continued for two years. When she fortified her diet with raw wheat germ, lecithin, brewer's yeast and other hair-nourishing foods her condition was rapidly on the mend.

In another case, a woman's daughter lost not only her hair but even her eyebrows a short time after taking reducing pills. For over three years she was without hair; during this time she had consulted a number of specialists but none was able to help. She finally agreed to follow her mother's suggestion of trying brewer's yeast and plenty of it, with the result that in about three months her eyebrows and all her hair had grown back.

FURTHER VALUABLE TIPS ON DIET

This hair-raising diet has worked for others. It may work for you. The foods to be used in this diet are richer than the refined, processed foods most people are in the habit of eating, so start out with one new food or supplement and gradually work up to the complete program.

Include such foods as these in your diet every single day: All lean meats, beef, liver, organ meats, fish and fowl (but no pork), eggs, green vegetables, green salads, root vegetables (this includes Irish and sweet potatoes, baked or boiled in their skins), dairy products, *solid* fruits in season and dried fruit, especially apricots, fresh unsalted nuts and vegetable oils. (The dried fruits are best obtained from health food stores.)

Eat as many of your vegetables raw as you can. Cooking and heating destroys their enzymes.

Eat a lot of cucumbers if they agree with you, as they promote growth of hair due to their content of silicon and sulphur.

Do not drink water with your meals. If possible, drink even your coffee about 20 minutes before meals, or two hours after.

List of foods to avoid particularly:

White sugar
White flour

All white flour products, such as macaroni, noodles, spaghetti, etc.
Packaged goods
Canned fruit
Cold cereals
Soft drinks
Pork
All pastry, unless baked at home with natural products.
If you use coffee, make it caffeine free. Stop smoking.

Food, supplements and vitamins that may be used to replace the things above:

Protein powder
Wheat germ—raw
Brewer's yeast
Desiccated liver
Sunflower seeds or sunflower seed meal
Lecithin
Kelp
Carrot juice
Vegetable oils
A natural multi-vitamin and mineral tablet
Natural vitamin A from fish liver oils
1,000 milligrams (mg.) of natural vitamin C every single day
Sea spray salt
Use honey for *all* sweetening

Every Nutrient Is Important

The rationale is to provide your body with every mineral, vitamin, amino acid and enzyme it needs because even a partial deficiency of almost any nutrient can cause the hair to fall out. For example:

• Dr. R. Gubner reports *(Arch. Derm. Syph.,* 64,668,1951) that persons deficient in folic acid often become bald, but the hair grows in again when the vitamin is given.

• Every fraction of the vitamin B complex is vital to hair growth, especially inositol, folic acid, and choline; men require about twice as much vitamin B as women do. Brewer's yeast, raw wheat germ and sunflower seeds are rich sources of B complex, and also contain protein and other important factors that contribute to hair and scalp health.

• A scientifically controlled experiment by researchers of the Department of Nutritional Science at the University of California proved that if a man in good health is deprived of protein his hair will show signs of severe atrophy and diseased pigmentation. Weight for weight the protein content of sunflower seeds is much greater than that of meat. Alfalfa is another rich, natural source of protein.

• Sometimes a lack of iodine in the diet will cause falling hair, dry skin, and thin, brittle nails. According to a news dispatch in the *New York Times,*[4] seaweed, rich in iodine, vitamins and minerals, had "staggering results" growing hair on dogs.

• According to Alfred W. McCann, food chemist, "The hair not only of human beings, but of all animals, requires silicon." Steel cut oats, cucumbers, raw wheat germ, sesame seeds and other seeds are among the many natural foods that provide silicon.

• Vitamin E has been shown to stimulate the growth of hair. Wheat germ oil, rich in vitamin E, has been used by mink growers to produce thick beautiful coats of fur on their animals.

• Vegetable oils are important for scalp health and hair growth due to the essential fatty acids they contain. These factors nourish the sebaceous glands which lubricate the hair and scalp. Animals become hairless if kept on diets lacking in unsaturated fatty acids.

To Sum Up

To state it briefly, there are hair and scalp-nourishing foods, and hair and scalp-starving foods; therefore what you eat or fail to eat largely affects your rate of hair loss or growth.

SUGGESTIONS FOR LOCAL TREATMENT

Can baldness be treated from the outside to any appreciable extent? The answer seems to be yes—in some cases.

A variety of plants and plant products have solid reputations for correcting certain conditions of thinning hair and barren scalps. While it is true that such folk remedies are regarded as unscientific, still many people who have tried them claim impressive results.

---

[4] February 11, 1965.

Perhaps we should keep in mind that the rich backlog of herbal lore covering many illnesses from bellyache to virus infection has led to the discovery of priceless herbal substances now developed into standard usage. On this basis, then, it is not unreasonable to suppose that when modern investigators look more diligently into folklore medication for baldness and falling hair they may discover that some of these remedies are founded on sound principles. As a matter of fact a few scientists here and there are already working along these lines, and so far the results of their experiments seem to indicate that certain plant constituents are effective in stimulating hair growth.

Vegetable Oils Applied

In an issue of *Prevention* magazine there was an article about vitamin E taken orally causing the hair to grow more quickly. The article ended with the query as to what would happen if vitamin E were rubbed directly on the scalp. In reference to this, a correspondent wrote: "The answer to that question was provided long ago by a man I know who has succeeded in growing hair on men and women by the application of a mixture of pure vegetable oils. First he thoroughly combs and brushes the hair. Then he applies the oil and massages it into the scalp until the scalp completely absorbs the oil. The hair on my scalp has been thinning out over the years, a condition prevalent with so many women. Not only has the process succeeded in stopping this loss but new hairs are gradually appearing and my scalp has never been healthier." [5]

Japanese Experiments with Vitamin E

Two Japanese researchers, Kamimura and Sasaki, of the Department of Dermatology, Sapporo Medical College, Japan, described experiments in which topical applications of vitamin E stimulated hair growth in test animals.

The dermatologists carefully shaved six identical circles, spaced one centimeter apart, on the backs of white male rabbits. Three different solutions were used to treat the shaved areas once a day:

---

[5] *Prevention*, September 1966.

natural vitamin E, synthetic vitamin E, and a solution of alcohol with five percent castor oil which was used as the control.

Every week 20 hairs were pulled from the circles and measured. Results of the test showed that the hairs treated with vitamin E grew 2.4 times faster than those of the control. During the early weeks the areas treated with natural vitamin E showed a slight but decided advantage over the areas receiving the applications of synthetic vitamin E.

Why Vitamin E Works

According to scientists the healthy activity of the hair bulb depends on a high energy production in the cells, and this in turn requires oxygen and glucose. Since it has been scientifically established that vitamin E protects the body's stores of oxygen, it is reasonable to expect that extra vitamin E on the hair bulb would stimulate hair growth.

Naturally we know that the health and growth of the hair do not depend on one factor alone. What the experiments of the Japanese researchers show is that if you are bald or losing your hair, vitamin E could be the one thing you are lacking. All types of lotions and tonics have been tried by men and women anxious to restore or keep their hair. Why not vitamin E? Wheat germ oil is a very rich source of vitamin E, or you can use vitamin E capsules.

The experiments conducted by the Japanese researchers ran from ten to 13 weeks. Rubbing the oil from one or two capsules of vitamin E daily into your scalp for that period of time is an inexpensive and safe baldness remedy well worth trying.

Herbalists' Treatment for Alopecia

Alopecia is a condition in which the hair suddenly falls out in patches. Medical herbalists treat alopecia by painting the bald spots with a mixture of two drams of bay leaf oil and one ounce of pure almond oil. This is also said to be effective for treating severe cases of dandruff.

Sarsaparilla—The Hair Strengthener of the Indians

The American Indians, as a rule, had strong thick hair. Back in the 18th century Le Page Du Pratz was requested by the U.S. government to make a special investigation of plants and their uses by the Indian tribes of the lower Mississippi Valley. In reporting on the virtues of sarsaparilla, he wrote: "It has that [virtue] of making the hair grow, the native women make use of it for this purpose with success. With this object they take the root, cut it into little pieces, boil it, and wash their hair in this water. I have seen many whose hair reached beyond the buttocks and one among them whose hair descended to the heels."

A few decades ago a medical doctor living in Mexico, where Jamaica sarsaparilla grows abundantly, discovered that the plant contains an important male hormone known as testosterone.

Many years later, during the 23rd annual meeting of the American Academy of Dermatology, Dr. Christopher M. Papa reported dramatic results in treating cases of baldness with a cream containing the male hormone. (Testosterone used in this preparation was obtained from animals, not sarsaparilla.) Hair began to grow after the cream was applied daily for several months to the scalps of balding male volunteers. One of the most successful treatments of the 16 out of 21 patients who achieved good results was that of a 78-year-old man, completely bald for 30 years.

Further investigation showed that testosterone was not creating new hair follicles. Dr. Papa explained that what seems to be a hairless scalp turns out to be covered with a very fine fuzz when subjected to microscopic examination. "There is hair present," he says, "but it is downy hair that is not visible. There is something to work on."

This hair-raising experiment remains an enigma because when testosterone is circulating within the blood stream it contributes to male pattern baldness. Why it acts differently when applied to the scalp is unknown.

Since testosterone itself can produce side effects, physicians are hesitant to prescribe the powerful hormone just to stimulate the growth of hair. But medics are hopeful that in the future a safe, synthetic male hormone will be developed.

In the meantime, you might try the Indian method of using a decoction of sarsaparilla root as a hair-wash. Sarsaparilla contains the important hair-growing hormone along with other constituents. Its use may or may not produce the same good results for you as it did for the Indians. But one thing is certain—a hair-wash of sarsaparilla is completely harmless.

Other Herbal Applications for the Scalp

1. People almost bald have reported growing hair by rubbing the oil from garlic perles well into the scalp every night.
2. Here is another popular folk remedy. Pour equal parts of olive oil and oil of rosemary into a bottle. Shake well and massage into the scalp night and morning.

OTHER METHODS OF LOCAL TREATMENT

Providing good circulation of blood to the scalp is one of the most important aspects of any program for improving the growth and quality of your hair. The tiny capillaries in the head must be supplied with a rich flow of blood in order to feed the hair roots. Therefore a good daily routine consisting of brushing and massaging should be employed.

Brushing

Brush the hair regularly, at least morning and night, and more often if time permits. Remember, use only a brush made of soft natural bristles.

Brush the hair in all directions, against the grain as well as with the grain. In other words, alternate the brush strokes working from the back of the head to the front, then front to back and up on the sides, then down. Brushing in all directions greatly stimulates the circulation.

Thin, weak hair should be brushed very gently at first, until it becomes more vigorous.

Massage

Massage the scalp carefully with the finger tips or the base of the palm every morning and evening for about ten minutes each time. Don't rub the scalp with the fingers. Instead, spread the fingers and place them firmly on an area of the scalp, moving the skin itself backwards and forwards, and in a circular motion so that the scalp will loosen up. Work from the back to the front, then from side to side. Do a really good job.

If you want to use a vibrator, get the type that fits over the back of your hand so that only the palm and fingers come in contact with your scalp and hair.

The Slant Board

Many people, including prominent movie stars, have reported good results in stopping hair loss by combining massage with the use of a slant board for 15 minutes twice a day.

One end of a large board, approximately six feet in length, is placed on a chair so that it has a rise of from one and a half to two feet. For comfort the board can be padded with a blanket or any other suitable material. By lying on the slant board with your feet at the high end, you cause the blood to flow down to your head, so while you are in this position your scalp is thoroughly massaged.

Those using the slant board generally start slowly, using the board for about five minutes at first, then gradually increasing the time each day until they work up to the full 15-minute periods.

HAIR CARE WITH HERBS AND HERBAL PRODUCTS

To make the switch from chemical hair preparations to nature's gentle products it is only necessary to take the first step, for there are wonderful herbs available which are safe to use and which are excellent promoters of scalp and hair health. Herbal shampoos, hair and scalp conditioners, wave-setting lotions, aromatic vinegars and hair tonics can easily be prepared right in your own home.

Herbal Shampoos

Dirt, dust, grime, and dandruff clog the roots of the hair and must be washed away, allowing the skin to breathe. The day before shampooing your hair rub a little warm olive oil gently but thoroughly into your scalp for ten minutes, working the skin backwards and forwards. This loosens the dandruff and dead residue.

For washing your hair, use shampoos made of natural herbs and herb oils. Be sure to rinse all the soap out of your hair but do not allow the full force of water to strike your head, as the shock weakens delicate hair. Instead apply a gentle steady stream of water from the faucet, or from an attachment that gives a soft spray. This requires a little patience but is well worth it.

To help keep soap out of the eyes when shampooing rub a little vaseline or cold cream across the forehead.

After shampooing your hair, blot it dry with a towel; never brush or rub it dry.

Recipes for Herbal Shampoos

1. Place a heaping teaspoonful each of nettle, rosemary, chamomile, mullein, and peach leaves in a porcelain or Pyrex bowl. Pour one pint of boiling water over the herbs, cover the bowl and allow the infusion to stand for 15 to 20 minutes. Strain and add shavings of castile soap while the liquid is still warm enough to dissolve them.

2. *Nature's Shampoo.* Soapwort herb, also commonly known as Bouncing Bet, is cultivated in gardens and found growing wild. It reaches a height of from two to four feet, and bears clusters of flowers varying in color from pink to white and purplish white. The herb was given the name soapwort because a strong soapy lather is produced when the leaves or chips of the bark are boiled in water. As a substitute for soap in shampoos it is excellent.

Boil four ounces of soap bark chips in one pint of distilled water. Boil very slowly until the liquid is reduced to one-half. Strain and bottle for use. You now have a preparation sufficient for several shampoos. The solution may be scented with a few drops of fragrant oil, such as oil of lavender or rosemary.

3. *Soapless Shampoos.* To one large or two small whole eggs beaten thoroughly, add two tablespoons of glycerine and six drops of almond oil. First brush your hair, then part the hair in sections approximately one-half inch wide and apply the mixture with the finger tips. When the entire scalp has been covered, comb the

mixture through the hair to the ends. Now massage the scalp and hair for ten minutes, then rinse thoroughly several times with warm water until the egg mixture is completely washed out. Do not use hot water as this coagulates the eggs.

Vinegar Rinse

A solution of vinegar and water is excellent for dissolving soap film which is sometimes difficult to rinse out of the hair. In addition to cutting the soap, it helps restore the normal acid mantle to the scalp. Normal skin is acid, while soap is alkaline. Soap shampoos cause the scalp to become temporarily alkaline, and it may take up to 24 hours before the normal acid condition returns to the scalp. A vinegar rinse neutralizes the alkaline effects of the soap and also serves as a mild antiseptic.

Use ¼ cup of vinegar to one quart of warm water. Pour slowly over the head. The vinegar rinse is used last, after the hair has been rinsed several times with plain water.

Aromatic Vinegar Rinses

A vinegar rinse may be scented by steeping with aromatic botanicals, or by adding a few drops of fragrant herbal oils.

Suggested combinations: Equal parts of rosemary, dried lavender flowers, cut orris roots.

Herb oils: Rosemary, bergamot, lavender, violet. Just a few drops of the oil are generally sufficient for each quart of vinegar.

Dry Shampoos

Dry shampoos are made of herbal powder which is dusted and massaged into the hair and scalp from a container with a perforated top. The powder is allowed to remain on the hair all night and is brushed out in the morning.

Two very fine dry herbal shampoos are made as follows:

1. Powdered orris roots—8 oz.
   Cassia buds (coarsely ground)—3 grams

   Mix together thoroughly and rub through a fine sieve. Use about once a week.

2. Powdered orris roots—1/2 oz.
   Corn starch—8 oz.
   Oil of violets—10 drops

   Mix and use in the same way as the first recipe.

Hair and Scalp Conditioners

Too much sun, harsh chemical shampoos and dyes, hair preparations that contain alcohol, or too frequent permanents are some of the things that rob the hair of its natural oils. The purpose of a hair conditioner is to replace these oils and add texture to your hair.

1. Mix the following herbal oils and rub gently into the scalp every two or three nights:

Sweet almond oil . . .	3 oz.
Rosemary oil	1 oz.
Lavender oil	30 drops

2. The scalp can be stimulated and the hair kept in good condition by the application of a little warm olive oil mixed with oil of marjoram.
3. Massage any vegetable oil or wheat germ oil thoroughly but gently into the scalp.
4. Orange-scented treatment for dry hair:

Oil of orange	20 drops
Sweet almond oil . . .	3 oz.
Rosemary oil	1 oz.

After a few weeks your hair should be much more attractive and softer to the touch.

Note: If your hair is already in a natural oily condition and a fragrance is desired, you can use any essential oil, such as oil of violet or lavender, but much more sparingly and only once a week.

To Keep the Hair in Place

Here is something you can use instead of chemical sprays for keeping your hair in place: Squeeze a little lemon juice into a small bowl and apply to the hair with a piece of cotton. It takes no more than a few minutes for the application to dry. Now brush your hair and you'll find that it will not only stay in place but will have a beautiful sheen. This simple lemon treatment also helps to highlight the waves of curly hair.

Hair Tonics

For hair that is dull, limp, lifeless looking or dry with frayed ends:

1. After you have shampooed your hair and before rinsing with vinegar, apply mayonnaise rich in vegetable oils, lemon juice and eggs. Work in gently over the entire head and allow to remain for one-half hour. Rinse thoroughly with warm water, shampoo lightly again and finish with a vinegar rinse.
2. Here is another: Beat one large egg into half a pint of water and add a few drops of rosemary oil. Gently massage the solution into the hair and scalp. Allow to remain for 15 minutes, then rinse thoroughly with warm water.
3. Tonic for faded hair: Mix one ounce of oil of rosemary and one ounce of coconut oil with three ounces of oil of sweet almonds. Rub a small amount of the oils gently into the scalp every other night.

Herbal Rinse for Very Fine, Unmanageable Hair

This type of hair is normal for some people. The slightest breeze disturbs its general shape; it also immediately flattens out under a head scarf or a snug-fitting hat.

Here are two excellent herbal rinses that will give more body to very fine, unmanageable hair:

1. Place a good handful of nettle leaves in a large Pyrex or porcelain bowl. Pour one quart of boiling water over the herb; cover and allow to steep until cool. Strain and pour over the head, using a second container to catch the liquid so that the hair may be rinsed several times. If the hair is put up in curlers directly following this rinse, it will comb out into strong fluffy waves.
2. Prepare an infusion of peach leaves or rosemary, and use in the same way as the nettle rinse.

Recipe for Getting Rid of Dandruff

Keep combs and brushes scrupulously clean. Brush the hair gently but thoroughly night and morning. Prepare the following lotion:

> Rosemary leaves—3 oz.
> Borax—3 tablespoonfuls
> Steep in 1 quart of boiling water.
> When cold, add:
> 30 drops of cologne
> 1/2 oz. of glycerine

Massage into the scalp gently once or twice a day.

Herbal Lotions for Setting Your Hair

1. A simple preparation is made as follows:

> Gum tragacanth . . . . ¾ oz.
> Rosewater . . . . 1 pint
> Sweet almond oil . . . ½ tsp.

Break the tragacanth into small pieces and soak in the rosewater. Allow to stand in a warm place, shaking the mixture occasionally until the gum is softened into a gelatine-like solution. Strain through a cloth, then add the oil and mix thoroughly. The preparation is then ready to use.

2. Here is another lotion:

> Carrageen moss . . . . 1 oz.
> Cologne spirits . . . . . 1 pint
> Orange flower water
> or rosewater . . . . 1 pint

Soak the carrageen moss in water over gentle heat until dissolved. Add cologne spirits, then strain and add the orange or rose water.

3. A third lotion uses quince seeds:

> Quince seeds . . . . . . 3 tsps.
> Hot water . . . . 1 pint
> Oil of lavender . . . . . 15 drops

The quince seeds must be soaked in the hot water for about three hours. Then strain and mix the liquid with the essential oil and cologne water.

CHAPTER SUMMARY

1. Your hair deserves the best of care, so don't subject it to harsh detergent shampoos or chemical preparations that can cause damage. Instead make your own hair-care solutions from safe gentle herbs.
2. Cleanliness is essential to the health of the scalp and hair. If your hair is dry, wash it once a week with an herbal shampoo, twice if it is oily.
3. To promote good circulation of blood to the scalp, massage and brush your hair every day. The practice of massaging may be combined with the use of a slant board.
4. Unrestricted use of salt in the diet has been linked to baldness so cut down on your intake of salt.
5. Local applications of certain plant solutions have been known to check hair fall and stimulate the growth of hair in some cases.
6. The do-it-yourself hair-growing program formulated by a modern nutritionalist who has researched the age-old problem of baldness may work for you, even if you have a "horseshoe" hairline.
7. In following the nutritional program you must switch to a type of diet which increases the reproductive potentials of the hair follicles and supplies the needed nutrients for new hair growth. Some of the foods suggested are wheat germ, wheat germ oil, sunflower seeds, pumpkin seeds, raw fruits and vegetables. And you might also include local applications of vitamin E to the hair and scalp.
8. The herbal hair care formulas in this chapter are all natural with no undesirable side-effects.

6

How Herbs Can Help Sharpen
Your Memory

"Allowing oneself to slip mentally as well as physically is the primary cause of deterioration," says Dr. William Kountz, director of Scientific Research of Gerontological Research Foundation, St. Louis, Missouri. "Memory loss is not a sign of aging," he adds, "but a sign of increasing carelessness."

He told of a patient 77 years old whose memory was failing. The patient had an opportunity to spend two years in Greece visiting his daughter, who had married a diplomat. However, since he couldn't speak a word of Greek he discovered it was almost impossible to find his way around the city. Out of necessity he diligently applied himself to the study of the language until he became proficient, and this mental discipline restored his memory. From then on he could remember the names, addresses, and even the phone numbers of all his friends, something he had been unable to do for some time.

"Keep your mind going," urges Dr. Kountz. "One, by constant activity, and two, by proper diet. The proper evaluation of the body from the standpoint of its chemistry is needed in order to supply the body with adequate food substances, such as minerals and vitamins and hormones—and proteins in particular."

HERBS AS MEMORY-AIDS

Can herbs also help you to function with a minimum of embarassing lapses of memory? In the opinion of the modern

107

medical herbalist the answer is "yes." Not content to render a healthful service to your body, certain herbs also "go to your head" and help you remember that important telephone number, and the name of the pretty blonde you wanted to introduce to Jim what's-his-name.

So let's take a stroll down memory lane and examine some of the best known of the numerous herbs that have reportedly helped many people to overcome a sluggish memory.

SAGE—FOR AGE

Almost everyone knows that sage *(Salvia officinalis)* is a popular culinary herb used especially in poultry dressings. What is not so well known however is that this herb has always played a great part in the history of botanic medicine. "Sage for old age" is a Chinese adage that apparently contains more truth than poetry. The herb has a centuries-old reputation as a sacred plant capable of exerting a beneficial influence on the brain, nerves, eyes, and glands. Gerard wrote that he found sage effective for "quickening the senses and memory, strengthening the sinews and restoring health to those suffering from palsies of moist cause, removing shaking and trembling of limbs."

What Sage Generally Contains

In pharmaceutical writings sage is listed among the natural antiseptics. It contains a volitile oil, resin, tannin, and a bitter principle. The oil is composed of camphor, salvene, cineol, and pinene. The fresh leaves provide appreciable amounts of vitamins A and C. (Vitamin A is generally regarded as the "eye vitamin.")

Modern Therapeutic Uses of Sage

Sage has been found to have an action on the cortex of the brain which is said to be beneficial in mental exhaustion, strengthening the ability to concentrate. It has also been found to insure relaxation in cases of general hypersensitivity and cerebrospinal irritation.

T. Bartram, F.N.I.M.H., writes glowingly of the therapeutic power of sage:

"Why am I so keen to get you interested in a plant reckoned to be good for nothing but stuffing? You've surely read of those Riders of the Purple Sage who were notorious for their rude health and full-blooded spirits? Well, in all probability some of the atomic sparkle of sage got under their skin. Didn't you know it had a long reputation for vitality—expecially in old age?

"Mr. J.B. had spent years at overwork, and the business stresses of an insurance agent had worn him out before his time. He was fit for the scrap-heap at 55—and he looked it. His harassed face was more lined that his father's at 80! His nerves were like those of a man perpetually handling a pneumatic drill, and the twitching of his eye never stopped. What else could he do? Insurance was the only thing he knew, and he was totally unable to hold down a job under present-day pressures. 'Rest—that's the only thing' advised his doctors. And he'd had months of that with little improvement.

"He went for a holiday in the south of England to help him relax, and there met a bank clerk who had cured himself of the same trouble with sage tea. He went into action at once. When he could not get a dozen fresh leaves to infuse in a teapot of boiling water he made a tea by using two heaped teaspoons of the dried culinary herb. One wineglassful after meals became a daily ritual for the following six months, after which he was able to pass his company doctor's examination and report for duty.

"But you do not have to be in as poor a condition as he to derive benefit. In the Middle Ages sage was known as 'Clear Eyes' because it cleared the vision and strengthened the eyes. Others have found it useful for catarrh, when prepared as above.

"A society of school teachers tried it out and many members declared it wonderfully strengthened the memory and seemed to clear the brain when tired.

"Maybe it is not without significance that the ancient Egyptians associated this plant with the spleen—an organ closely related to some of those obscure psychological patterns thrown up by this schizophrenic age."

MUGWORT—AN HERBAL BRAIN TONIC

Beifuss. - Besenkraut.

Mugwort *(Artemisia vulgaris)* is a species of wormwood but can be distinguished from its more popular relative *(Artemisia absin-*

thium) by the color and shape of its leaves which are green above and whitish underneath, with sharply pointed segments.

Mugwort is employed extensively in Chinese medicine, and is also used in China as a charm during the Dragon Festival when it is hung up in the main room of the home. At one time mugwort was so highly venerated in that country that the Chinese rebel Huang Ch'ao instructed his soldiers to spare the lives of anyone in whose home the herb was found.

Modern Uses

Modern herbalists classify the therapeutiac action of mugwort as tonic, nervine, stimulant, diaphoretic, and emmenagogue. C.F. Leyel says: "The connection between the brain and the spinal cord is so intimate that herbs which affect the spine are likely to have an action on some part of the brain . . . mugwort for instance, stimulates the spinal cord and relieves congestion in the brain. . . . Sleep walking is often combatted by mugwort. It is a good brain tonic."

Note: Mugwort tea may be prepared from the dried leaves or dried blossoms. Made exclusively from the blossoms, and flavored with honey, the tea offers a unqiue and highly pleasant taste.

ROSEMARY–THE HERB OF REMEMBRANCE

Rosemary *(Rosmarinus officinalis)* is another herb that has long been used to clear the cobwebs from the memory. The Greeks and Romans prepared a fragrant distilled water from the flowers and inhaled the odor so that "the evils were destroyed from the mind and the memory no longer played tricks." Dr. James wrote: "Rosemary is a plant of great service in affections of the head and nerves. . . . It strengthens the sight and memory."

At one time many of the French hospitals used the herb to deodorize sickrooms and to prevent the spread of infection. This is quite interesting as today we find rosemary oil listed among the active ingredients of two modern germicide sprays sold in drug stores.

Mystically, rosemary symbolizes loyalty, love, and immortality, and it was once believed to strengthen the heart as well as the memory.

Modern Uses

Today, rosemary is still regarded as an antidote to mental fatigue and forgetfulness. A tisane (tea) of the herb is becoming popular with tired businessmen and students who find it refreshing and a good natural remedy for bringing added agility to the intellect.

Dr. Eric Powell informs us that tests over a lengthy period of time have demonstrated that there's a lot to the old saying, "Rosemary—that's for remembrance." He says: "There is no doubt that small doses of fresh rosemary help improve the memory. In common with camomile and wild yam, it is also of much service in the treatment of congested headaches and insomnia. It undoubtedly has an affinity for the brain."

A Staunch Supporter of Rosemary for Memory

When asked how she managed to retain such a keen, alert memory at 88 years of age, Mrs. D.B. replied: "I don't know what all the fuss is about—so many people asking about my memory. In the little village where I grew up, everyone young and old drank rosemary tea every day. Why, I thought folks everywhere in the world knew that rosemary was good for the memory." With that she pointed toward a row of bushes in her yard. "That's all rosemary," she said. "I planted that myself years ago when I moved here. I wouldn't dream of being without my rosemary tea!"

EYEBRIGHT—HERBAL MEMORY REVIVER

Since eyebright herb *(Euprasia officinalis)* is widely recognized among herbalists as a specific for certain eye disorders, few people know that the plant also has a reputation as a first class memory reviver. Several physicians have reportedly praised the therapeutic value of eyebright in memory training and in strengthening of the mental faculties. For example, Dr. Asuda, a Japanese physician, claimed that he had successfully treated over 500 patients troubled with faulty memory, by administering eyebright.

Mr. K.R. writes: "In my own work I have frequently derived therapeutic benefit from infusing one ounce of eyebright in one and a half pints of boiling water, adding two tablespoonfuls of clover honey, sieving when cold, and drinking a wineglassfull between meals; the result being the ability to remember facts and incidents—including those best forgotten!"

GARLIC—NATURE'S BULB TO LIGHT THE MEMORY LAMP

Even the lowly garlic bulb has been credited with keeping the memory lamp burning brightly well into advanced years. This humble herb has had the distinction of being used by no less a prominent personage than a president's wife. Back in 1959 when the late Mrs. Eleanor Roosevelt reached the age of 75, the *Chicago Daily News* covered the event and commented on the excellent health of the former First Lady, stating that "she is still going full-steam ahead at such a clip that she leaves persons less than half her age gasping for breath."

It was pointed out that Mrs. Roosevelt exercised regularly and also that "she takes vitamin pills and three chocolate-coated garlic pills recommended by her doctor to stimulate her memory, which she says has never been anything to 'brag' about."

YERBA MATÉ—EXOTIC MEMORY BEVERAGE
OF SOUTH AMERICA

Among the South Americans, yerba maté (pronounced mah-tay) is the tea *par excellence* for its bracing and tonic effect on mind and body. They drink the beverage at mealtimes and also throughout the day. It is very popular with all classes—the elite, the gauchos or cowboys of the pampas (plains), and the natives, especially those doing heavy manual labor.

This small, thickly branched evergreen tree is known botanically as *Ilex paraguayensis* and is a member of the holly family. It grows wild in the river forests of Paraguay and southern Brazil; however it is also extensively cultivated in other areas of South America. It is estimated that the inhabitants of that continent consume approximately 8,000,000 pounds of yerba maté every year. The herb is also exported to the United States and other countries.

A Remarkable Tonic

A news article entitled "Paraguay, the Land of Fruit and Music" stated in part: "The national beverage of Paraguay is made of the plant maté, brewed as a substitute for ordinary Chinese, Ceylon, or Indian tea. This beverage effects a surprising rejuvenation of the human organism. One drinking it, especially the first time, feels a remarkable inflow of strength, energy, and cheerfulness, as a direct and almost immediate result. The natives of Paraguay cannot say too much in praise of its beneficial effects."

Maté Popular with the Missionaries as "Jesuit's Tea"

The early Jesuit missionaries learned the use of yerba maté from the Indians and found the brew so refreshing and healthful that they risked their lives searching for the small trees in the dense jungles of Brazil. Later they brought the tree under cultivation near their missions and maté became widely known as "Jesuit's tea" or "missionaries' tea." It was the Jesuits who added the word *yerba* (herb) to the Indian name *maté* which comes from a word meaning "drinking vessel" or "gourd." Long before the arrival of the white men, the Indians dried and powdered maté leaves and placed them in a water-filled gourd bowl, then dropped hot stones into the water to infuse the powder. The refreshing tea was then sipped through a tube or reed called a *bombilla,* as the Indians maintained that contact with the air caused the herb to lose much of its delicious flavor.

The white men used a similar technique for drinking yerba maté. They placed the powdered leaves in a bowl, poured on boiling water, then drank the tea through a tube, the lower end of which was fashioned into a sort of bulbous tea-strainer.

How a 75-Year-Old Man Recovered Failing Memory with Help from Yerba Maté

A 75-year-old widower, living with his son, daughter-in-law, and grandchildren, was slipping mentally. Grandpa could not remember their names or the names of his friends even though he saw his friends quite often. It was also necessary to lead him to the bathroom because he could never find it by himself.

On the advice of a friend, the family bought a bottle of dolomite tablets (a combination of magnesium, the "memory mineral," and calcium) and gave grandpa two of the tablets. Grandpa promptly spit them out. Coaxing, pleading, even bribing proved useless.

One day the son came across an article on yerba maté and learned that the herb contained many valuable constituents, including magnesium. He immediately went out and bought a pound of the herb tea. Much to his delight, grandpa loved yerba maté and drank it every day.

Then early one morning about a month later, the son heard a noise and got up to see what it was. To his amazement, grandpa, all by himself, was just coming out of the bathroom. "Shame on you, son, for staying in bed so late," the old man chided. "Guess I'll have to make my own herb tea this morning." With that he shuffled into the kitchen and began humming as he filled the teapot with water.

Encouraged by the startling progress the old man was making, the family got out the bottle of dolomite in hopes of helping things along. Again grandpa promptly spit out the tablets. This time the family had a strong bargaining point—no dolomite, no yerba maté. Grandpa took the dolomite: two tablets three times a day. A few more supplements such as lecithin and wheat germ oil were gradually added to the old man's diet.

Three months later, much to the joy of the family, grandpa's memory had improved dramatically. He could easily remember all the names of his relatives and friends, and even that of the neighbor down the block. The return to more youthful attributes were obvious in other ways, too. He was cheerful, energetic, and took an active and lively interest in the world around him.

Therapeutic Actions of Yerba Maté

Medical authorities of South America who have carefully studied yerba maté have drawn the following conclusions regarding the effects of this unique herb:

- It is a general stimulant both to the intellect and the body, yet its stimulating power does not interfere with sleep.
- It is a tonic to the brain, nerves, and spine, and has a strengthening effect on the memory.
- It helps prevent infection and also indigestion.
- It aids urinary and fecal evacuations.
- It is a general antiscorbutic and body builder.
- It increases respiratory power.
- It is an excellent febrifuge.
- It lessens the sensation of hunger.
- It nourishes the smooth tissues of the intestines.
- It is not a drug, but a food.

Constituents of Yerba Maté and Their General Health Value and Memory Power

Clues to the effectiveness of yerba maté as a health beverage lie in the plant's constituents.

Yerba maté is rich in vitamin C, and also provides natural mineral salts—magnesium, calcium, iron, sodium, potassium, manganese, silica, and phosphates. In addition it yields an alkaloid known as *Mattein.*

Vitamin C prevents scurvy, and also fights general infection. One of the first symptons of *vitamin C* shortage is "pink toothbrush" or the appearance of black and blue marks from a slight bruise. This vitamin helps prevent bleeding into the tissues, bleeding gums, irritability, tiredness, and painful cracks at the corners of the mouth.

The relation between a lack of *vitamin C* and senile dementia (including loss of memory) is apparent from the following report in a scientific journal:

> A senile patient is forgetful, confused, his speech rambles. He repeats a question that has just been answered. Memory is so poor the individual does not recognize members of his own family.
>
> Dr. Berkenau made a study of "senile dementia" patients at the Warneford Hospital, Oxford, England, in 1940. He found all his patients were short of vitamin C. No exceptions. "A deficit of 1500 milligrams may be regarded as pathological (disease causing)." The deficit of these patients varied from 2400 to 3000 milligrams.

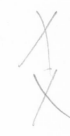

"Plaques appeared in the brain of senile patients identical to those found in alcoholics. This indicates a poisonous origin. Hence senile patients and those approaching old age need substantial quantities of vitamin C to protect their brain from damage and to fight infections."

Along with *vitamin C,* we note that yerba maté also contains *calcium,* the mineral necessary for the health of the muscles and nerves and for regulating the rhythm of the heart beat. A shortage of *calcium* can make you tense, irritable, or give you muscle cramps or insomnia. *Sodium,* which nature has added to yerba maté, helps keep *calcium* in solution. A deficiency of sodium may cause intestinal and stomach gases. *Potassium,* another mineral present in the small Brazilian tree, helps the kidneys to eliminate waste products from the body. It works with *sodium* to nourish the muscular system. A shortage of *potassium* may cause insomnia, nervousness, constipation, gas formation, muscle weakness, poor breathing, fatigue, and irregular heart beat. *Iron* is essential for the formation of rich red blood.

Magnesium is the "memory mineral," and is sometimes called the "mineral of life," so vital is its importance to your entire being. This precious mineral which is contained in yerba maté can spell the difference between the sluggish, foggy mentality typical of senility, and the performance of quick, alert, well-coordinated brain and muscle power typical of youth.

And we find that *magnesium* also helps to maintain normal blood pressure, that it speeds the healing process, that it helps to dissolve or prevent kidney stones, and that it helps lower cholesterol. The motor nerves are dependent on *magnesium* for proper transmission of nerve impulses from brain to muscles.

When we consider that all these precious constituents and more are present in yerba maté, it is not surprising that the beverage produces such healthful effects!

Note: Yerba maté is prepared like ordinary tea—about one teaspoonful to a cup of boiling water. Honey or lemon may be added to taste. When iced, it makes a refreshing and delightful summer drink.

CHAPTER SUMMARY

1. The older we get the more essential it becomes for us to keep active, as withdrawal of either mind or muscle can result in atrophy.
2. Proper nutrition supplemented with herbs, along with keeping the mind constantly active, are vital keys to preserving or regaining memory power.
3. Select herbs are powerful energizers which can help us to function with a minimum of embarassing memory lapses.
4. In addition to producing an invigorating effect on the memory, specific herbs also render a valuable service to the health of the body.
5. Nature offers a wide selection of herbs to choose from to please the individual taste and to aid in maintaining mental vigor and vitality.
6. Yerba maté is a veritable storehouse of valuable constituents, including magnesium—the "memory mineral."

7

Herbal Preparations to Help You Sleep

Some insomniacs count sheep in an effort to tranquilize their overactive minds; others pray to the Good Shepherd: "Now I lay me down to sleep—I hope."

But the majority of sleepless Americans seek material help for eyes that will not close or stay closed at bedtime. Hundreds of millions of dollars a year are spent on various devices to help the insomniac find the path to slumberland—eye shades, ear plugs, specially designed pillows and mattresses, twinkling luminous objects, and even special phonograph records of rhythmic, tranquilizing sounds. Whether any of these things do much good only the user knows for sure, but at least they do no harm.

On the other hand, insomnia has led a legion of hollow-eyed sufferers to drug-taking for wooing the sandman. An estimated 15 million sleeping pills are swallowed by Americans every night. In England and Wales the number of prescriptions for barbituates, sedatives, and hypnotics amounts to one-quarter of the total number of prescriptions filled.

According to a report by the U.S. Public Health Service, more accidental deaths result from an excess of barbituates than from any other type of acute drug poisoning. Continued use of sleep-inducing drugs sometimes brings about a trance-like state rather than genuine sleep. In these instances the insomniac cannot remember exactly how many tablets he has already swallowed so he takes more. This puts him to sleep for good. In other cases people make the serious and often fatal blunder of taking sleeping pills just before or shortly after drinking liquor. Fatalities caused by this practice are not uncommon. In analyzing 21 deaths caused by alcohol and barbiturate poisoning, two British pathologists concluded that the combination acts tremendously fast to produce a fatal drop in blood pressure.

Varied Sleep Habits

Chronic insomnia occurs in various ways. Some people find it extremely difficult to fall asleep when they first get to bed. They toss and turn half the night and lose even more sleep worrying about not sleeping and wondering how they are going to get through the day when it comes time to get up. The second type falls asleep easily but wakes up abruptly after two or three hours and can't seem to get back to sleep again. Still another type snoozes soundly for a few hours but awakens with the roosters and remains awake until the alarm goes off. To others sleep comes only in fitful snatches—a beeping cycle of sleep-wake, sleep-wake.

Then there are the problems of snoring and nocturnal teeth grinding. The millions of people who fall into each of these classes sleep well enough themselves in spite of their noisy imitations of buzz saws or grinding cement mixers. But pity the unfortunate sleeping partner! Snoring and toothgrinding habits have caused many a spouse to seek a separate bedroom or threaten divorce in response to too many sleepless nights.

Seven Levels of Sleep

A research project on sleep, conducted at Cornell University and reported in the *British Medical Journal*,[1] indicates that there are seven levels or planes of sleep, which are distinguised as follows:

(1) A period of wakefulness in which conversation is possible and the subject, although at physical rest, still responds to external stimuli by conscious attention. (2) A period of pre-sleep in which muscular relaxation is greater than in plane 1, fantasy life is enriched, drowsiness is obvious, and periods of dozing and transitory lack of awareness are common. The subject often feels some sensations of floating and depersonalization; subjective warmth permeates his body. (3) A period of light sleep in which objective response to stimuli occurs but is relatively unconscious, considerable muscular activity being

[1]March 1952.

present as further progressive relaxation of the many muscle groups is sought. (4) A period of heavy deep sleep in which little muscular movement is apparent, no response to external stimuli takes place, and the subject is "dead to the world." Wakefulness, in like fashion, is a reversal of the process of sleep and its passage contains a similar number of stages starting with deep sleep, although the time intervals are somewhat displaced. Plane 5 is the period of light sleep following deep sleep; plane 6, the period of pre-wakefulness; and plane 7, the actual awakening to the new world of tomorrow.

If we understand these different levels we will realize that in the stages of semi-wakefulness we are partly asleep and reaping the benefits of sleep. So if you have occasional bouts of sleeping poorly when first getting to bed, don't worry too much about it. Just keep in mind that in a few minutes you will be in the first stages of semi-wakefulness even though you may not be aware of it.

And some people who understand the gradual stages we go into before we have fully dropped off to sleep are content to remain in the second phase for a while and will not allow themselves to be disturbed out of it. For it is in the second pre-sleep state that fantastic ideas, visions, or messages often occur which are not idle senseless dreams. This strange phenomenon has been known for thousands of years. The ancient Egyptians and Greeks slept in sacred places in hopes of having dreams that would provide answers to their problems. And even in our own day many people pray for dreams of guidance when they prepare for sleep. The famous artist John Hulberg says that he gets many of his ideas from the "preconscious, the half-remembered, half-conscious things you see just before you fall asleep or wake up."

Is Too Much Salt Keeping You Awake?

Practically every insomniac is fully acquainted with the multitude of suggestions that have been offered to help him sleep: try to relax; leave your problems outside the bedroom; think pleasant thoughts; do some breathing exercises; sleep with your head to the north and your feet to the south; avoid noise, etc. But so far little has been said about the relation between sleep and dietary habits.

Some foods have a tranquilizing effect while others such as

coffee "rev up" your motor and block the way to slumberland. Salt is another sleep-thief as it stimulates the adrenal glands just as coffee does. After thousands of laboratory tests and five years of study on the problem of insomnia, a French doctor announced: "Cut out salt from your meals after mid-day, then you stand a very good chance of peaceful sleep."

American medics have also found salt to be an enemy of restful slumber. In addition to stimulating the adrenal glands, salt can lead to high blood pressure, a condition that makes sleep difficult by causing the temples to throb as the blood pounds its way through the veins. And since treatment usually calls for a diuretic, the patient is awakened frequently during the night by the urge to urinate.

In the *Journal of the American Medical Association*,[2] Dr. Michael Miller reported that he was able to help insomniacs who had been sleeping only one or two hours a night by simply putting them on a low-salt diet. Seventeen out of 20 patients began sleeping better almost immediately and by the end of three weeks were getting eight hours of sleep every night.

The Hidden Salt in Your Diet

Keep in mind that many foods are already salted, so if you decide to cut down on your sodium intake you must do more than just put aside your salt shaker. According to Dr. Snively, the average daily diet contains from five to 25 times as much salt (about 5000 mgs.) as people need for their well-being. Some examples of high sodium foods include ham, bacon, sausage. frankfurters, salami, pickles, relish, shell fish, meat soups, canned vegetables, sauerkraut, spinach, kale, olives, salted crackers, bread, pretzels, salted peanuts, potato chips, gravies, sauces, and all salted cheeses. Soft water also has a high sodium content.

The vital food salts we need for our well-being are provided naturally by fresh fruits, vegetables, fish, cereals, and meat. One cup of beets, for example, contains 220 milligrams of sodium, turnip greens 20, dandelion greens 152, carrots 62, kale 200; 3 1/2 ounces of turkey provides 40 milligrams, and the same amount of chicken breast will give you 78.

[2] September 22, 1945.

Calcium and Healthful Sleep

Certain herbs and foods contain valuable nutrients which help promote healthful sleep. For example, the body requires a continual supply of calcium for building bones, strengthening the muscles, and controlling the impulses that are transmitted through the nerves. In calcium deficiency the nerves are denied the basic material needed to quiet them down. As a result you feel jumpy and experience what is commonly called "a case of the nerves." Unless the demands are met, when you lie down to sleep there won't be enough calcium in your bloodstream to reach your brain and quiet the signals that are keeping you awake.

During the change of life, many women suffer sleepless nights. According to some researchers the sex hormones apparently play an important role in the bone-building process. When the sex hormones diminish as they do during and after the menopause, a plentiful supply of calcium is required so that the blood can deliver enough of it to satisfy all your body's needs, thereby preventing fragile bones, nervousness, and insomnia.

Natural Sources of Calcium

How much calcium do you require to help attract the comforting embrace of Morpheus, the god of sleep? Nutritionalist Adelle Davis suggests two grams of calcium every day. Calcium can be taken in tablet form, or you can get it by fortifying your diet with calcium-rich herb teas such as alfalfa, nettle, or motherwort. Alfalfa is also available in other forms—tablets, ground meal, sprouts, and "alfalfa fudge." Leafy green vegetables, soybeans, sunflower and sesame seeds are also abundant plant sources of calcium. Three ounces of sesame seeds contain 1,125 milligrams of calcium, whereas one glass of milk contains only 300 mgs.

Pantothenic Acid—the Vitamin That Aids Sleep

Pantothenic acid, commonly called the anti-stress vitamin, is another valuable substance for anyone who has trouble falling asleep. The daily requirement of pantothenic acid appears to be more than 50 milligrams a day, yet most people only get an average of three to five milligrams per day. This is not too surprising when we realize that this member of the vitamin B family is easily destroyed by heat, which means it is lost in the overcooking and canning process.

Herbs and other foods rich in pantothenic acid include wheat germ, brewer's yeast, green vegetables, whole grains, sunflower and sesame seeds, mushrooms, chickpeas, brown rice, egg yolk, beef, liver, heart, kidney, and the dark meat of chicken and turkey. Pantothenic acid is also available in tablet form.

Nocturnal [During Sleep] Tooth Grinding

Two nutrients, calcium and pantothenic acid, have been found helpful in curbing the habit of nocturnal tooth grinding. Calcium is urgently needed by the muscles, as a lack of this mineral will cause cramps or convulsions.

A convulsion is defined as "a violent involuntary series of contractions of the voluntary muscles." In medical jargon, the condition of gnashing or grinding the teeth is called *bruxism* ("an involuntary movement of the muscles of the mouth, bringing the teeth together in a grinding movement").

According to the Swiss dental scientist, Peter Schaerer: "The primary causes of bruxism seem to be changes in central nervous activity, as in sleep, in states of nervous tension, or in conflict situations. Psychological studies have shown that persons suffering from bruxism frequently display emotional disorders such as excessive fright or aggression, irritability, and tenseness." According to a report[3] by E. Cheraskin, M.D., D.M.D., and W.M. Ringsdorf, Jr., D.M.D., M.S., tooth grinding is a neuro-muscular problem that "should vanish in parallel with an increase in calcium consumption." The two Alabama researchers point out that in a multiple testing program which they set up, the subjects who stopped bruxing had increased their intake of calcium and the anti-stress vitamin, pantothenic acid.

In short, if your're grinding your teeth, your stresses are showing. And stress depletes the stores of pantothenic acid in the body.

---

[3]*Dental Survey,* 1970.

Handling the Problem of Snoring

During sleep the muscles relax, and if the muscle tone is weak the palate slackens and drops. This partially blocks the air passage, and the vibration of air against the barrier causes snoring. Children or young people rarely snore as their muscle tone is much firmer than that of a person middle-aged or older.

Based on the idea that snoring usually takes place when the individual sleeps flat on his back, a popular folk-remedy suggests that a small rubber ball be tied to the pajamas or night gown in the area between the shoulder blades. Then if the sleeper rolls on his back, the discomfort immediately causes him to turn over on his side again. But it seems to us that since the problem of snoring is one of weak muscle tone, an increase in the consumption of calcium (the muscle building mineral) would be the most sensible and helpful approach to alleviating the problem.

HERBAL SLEEP-AIDS

In olden times, long before the advent of sleeping pills, people used nature's gentle herbs for coping with insomnia. Herb teas, herbal baths, and herbal scent-therapy were folk remedies of the day. In the latter case, bedding was scented with a select fragrant botanical such as lavender, pine, camphor, hops, lime flowers, or orange blossoms. Even the famous artist Van Gogh used a plant substance for dealing with his problem of sleeplessness. He said, "I treat my insomnia with a very strong dose of camphor in my pillow and mattress."

Many centuries of experience have confirmed the value of soothing botanicals. The modern medical herbalist is still able to treat cases of insufficient sleep successfully, using the same plant formulas as did his earlier counterpart, but of course with the added advantage of research and modern methods of preparation.

Following is a collection of herbal remedies for insomnia which have remained constant over the ages.

HERBAL TEAS TO HELP YOU SLEEP

The beneficial effects of herb teas are said to be cumulative. In other words you may not get immediate results, but if you continue using the tea faithfully, after a few days you should begin sleeping better. Herbalists also point out that since there are different causes of insomnia, a specific herb tea may help one person and not another. Therefore it is best to select one herbal formula and try it for four or five consecutive days. In this way you will be able to find the remedy appropriate to your need.

BALM *(Melissa officinalis)*

Synonyms: Lemon balm, sweet balm, balsam, melissa.
Part Used: The herb.

Balm is native to France but naturalized in the United States and England. It grows in fields, along roadsides, and is well known as a garden plant. In its fresh state it has a strong lemony aroma, and was used as a strewing herb back in the days when scented botanicals were spread on bare floors.

The botanical name *melissa* is from the Greek word for honey. Bees are particularly fond of this plant. Among the ancient Greeks it was a practice to place sprigs of balm in bee hives to attract a swarm.

A cold infusion of balm taken freely is reputed to be excellent for its calming influence on the nerves. One ounce of the herb is placed in one pint of cold water and allowed to stand for 12 hours. The infusion is then strained and taken in small wineglassful doses throughout the day.

CHAMOMILE *(Matricaria chamomilla)*

Synonyms: German chamomile.
Part Used: The blossoms.

German chamomile has enjoyed a well-established reputation as a remedy for soothing the nerves and assisting digestion. In European countries the tea is a favorite beverage to take before retiring to assure a good night's sleep.

Chamomile is widely accepted as a domestic remedy for the treatment of nightmare and restless sleep, especially in children. Dr. Schall, an English physician, stated that the tea was effective both as a treatment and preventive of these complaints. For children, the usual infusion (prepared as ordinary tea) is taken in doses of one or two tablespoons three or four times a day. For adults, three or four cups a day are taken.

LADY'S SLIPPER *(Cypripedium pubescens)*

Synonyms: Nerve root, yellow moccasin, American valerian.
Part Used: The root.

This plant is an aromatic perennial that reaches from four to 28 inches in height. It has large yellow sac-like "slippers."

Medical herbalists regard lady's slipper as one of the best and safest nervines in the plant kingdom. Many of the old-time family physicians advised the use of this herb for nervous irritability and sleeplessness. The following excerpts are from a typical prescription of those times:

Lady's Slipper
Part Used: The root.

The medicine is an excellent nervine, and acts as a tonic to the exhausted nervous system. Hence it is adapted to cases of nervous irritability and sleeplessness, and gives rest and refreshing sleep and for this purpose is one of the best among domestic remedies.

Whenever a mild and safe nervine is needed, lady's slipper root is very generally used in the form of an infusion, made by steeping about one ounce of the root in a pint of boiling water. Dose, from a half to a teacupful every hour or two, or oftener, according to symptoms.

It was also pointed out that a fluid extract of the plant may be used "in doses of 15 to 25 drops."

Here is a much stronger form in which the herb is employed in many parts of the world: Three ounces of the cut root are placed in 12 ounces of cold distilled water and allowed to stand for two hours. When the time period is up, the decoction is brought to a boil and simmered for 15 minutes. The herb is then strained off and the liquid boiled again slowly until it is reduced to a half-pint. It is then bottled and stored in the refrigerator. This herbal preparation will not keep more than two or three days, when a fresh brew must be prepared again. For nervousness, one tablespoonful is taken in a wineglass of water three or four times a day. One tablespoonful in warm water is taken at bedtime to help promote drowsiness.

LIME FLOWERS *(Tilia europaea)*

Synonyms: Lindenflowers, Linden tree.
Part Used: The flowers.

The Germans were especially fond of the linden tree and named one of their streets in Berlin *Unter den Linden—* "under the linden."

The fragrance of lime flowers has a relaxing and soothing effect. It is said that even to sit under a lime tree in bloom causes drowsiness.

Lime flowers are used in the form of an infusion, one teaspoonful to one cup of boiling water. This is covered and allowed to stand for 15 minutes, then strained. One teaspoonful of honey is added and the lime-flower tea taken warm, not hot, just before bedtime.

One man who suffered from insomnia for four and a half years claimed that he had his first night of unbroken sleep after he gave up coffee and started drinking lime-flower tea. He also took five brewer's yeast tablets at meal times.

PASSIONFLOWER *(Passiflora incarnata)*

Synonyms: Passion vine, maypop, maypop herb.
Part Used: Plant, leaves, flowers.

This graceful and handsome climber is regarded as a mystical plant traditionally associated with the crucifixion. In its native habitat (Southern U.S. and the West Indies) it often climbs to the highest treetops and sends out an abundance of radiant white and purple flowers.

Passiflora is an ancient herbal sedative, nervine and antispasmodic which is still in use today. Dr. Leclerc of Paris showed that the herb had a calming effect on nervous restlessness. Many years of experiments have demonstrated that its use results neither in depression nor in disorientation.

R. Swinburne Clymer, M.D., recommends passionflower in cases of extreme nervousness and lack of sleep. He says, "It is quieting and soothing to the nervous system. The Nature physician refuses to give drugs that are habit forming. Passiflora takes the place of narcotics." Dr. Clymer suggests the following combination for insomnia:

Tincture Scutellaria (Scullcap) .... 1 oz.
Tincture Passiflora (Passionflower) .... 1 oz.
Dose, 20 to 60 drops in water as required.

For sleepless nights, T.C. Taws, Medical Herbalist of England, advises a mixture of one-half ounce each of passionflower, valerian, and hops added to one pint of boiling water. The container is immediately removed from the burner and the infusion allowed to stand for a few hours. "Strain, then take a wineglassful half an hour before retiring." Taws adds, "Encourage natural sleep with natural remedies and you'll awake the next day feeling brighter."

Three More Natural Beverages for Coping with Insomnia

1. Many people claim that a glass of warm milk laced with two teaspoons of honey is a remarkably effective nightcap.
2. Another old-fashioned remedy for sleeplessness is lettuce tea. Two or three of the outer leaves are thoroughly washed, then simmered for 20 minutes in one-half pint of water. This is strained and drunk hot just before bedtime.
3. A correspondent wrote: "I was looking for something that would help me sleep nights and this I found among the pages of old almanacs. Take a half-teaspoon of marjoram in one cup of hot milk at bedtime. It is very soothing. Here I have had marjoram in the house for some time and didn't know what it was for. Have been taking it for some time and find it so wonderful; I can now enjoy a good night's rest. Also have been telling some people who take sleeping pills to try it. How simple and good it is!"

HERBAL BATHS TO HELP YOU SLEEP

The old-fashioned herbal bath is a pleasant way to help sooth jangled nerves and calm a turbulent mind. Here are some of the herbs which may be employed:

Lady's slipper	Scullcap	Birch leaves
Lime flowers	Valerian	Passionflower
Hops	Catnip	Mugwort
Melissa	Rosemary	Khus-khus
Chamomile	Pine needles	Marigold
Lavender	Meadowsweet	Lovage

Herbal baths are simple to prepare. Just add four ounces of the botanical to a gallon of boiling water. Cover and simmer for ten to 15 minutes, then strain and add the decoction to the warm bath water. (You may use a single herb or prepare a mixture of two or three from those given on the list.)

Other Methods

1. Place the herb, or combination of herbs, in a cheesecloth bag. Tie with a piece of string to the spout of the bathtub, then turn the water on.
2. A cloth bag may be filled with the herbs, then tied securely and placed right in the tub.

Tips for Successful Herbal Baths

- Keep in mind that the purpose of the herbal bath is to help you relax so you can sleep when you get to bed. So take your regular bath or shower after you get home from work, and use the herbal bath just before bedtime.
- Herbal bathing should be done in a leisurely manner, so don't rush it. Soak in the tub for 15 or 20 minutes, gently massaging the muscles from time to time.
- The temperature of the bath should be comfortably warm, not hot. Hot baths, with or without the addition of herbs, cause the veins to become enlarged and a sense of heaviness is felt in the head, leaving the bather fatigued and weak.
- Some people find that the relaxing effects of the herbal bath are greatly enhanced when followed by drinking a cup of tranquilizing herb tea such as lime flower or lady's slipper, chamomile, etc.

THE HOP PILLOW—NATURE'S MAGIC SLEEP-AID

Hop-pickers of yesteryear claimed that the strong odor of hops produced drowsiness. And even in modern times many instances have occurred in which people entering an "oast house" where hops were being dried experienced such a profoundly tranquilizing effect that they were compelled to sit down and soon found themselves in a deep, refreshing sleep!

Back in the old days people took advantage of the sedative fragrance of the plant, and a pillow stuffed with hops was used in place of an ordinary pillow as a soothing sedative in conditions of insomnia. This folk-practice was regarded as superstitious nonsense until a physician prescribed a hop pillow for King George III in 1787 with excellent results. It is also a matter of record that a hop pillow was used with the greatest success by the Prince of Wales in 1879.

Hop Pillow a Remarkable Sleep-Aid

The hop pillow has proved to be of remarkable value for tense, nervous people who are unable to sleep. Scientific research has shown that hops contain certain substances which act as a sedative in overcoming insomnia. Lupulin, the active principle, has been used with good effect in war psychosis.

In the 17th edition of the *U.S. Dispensatory* we read:

> A pillow of hops has proved useful in allaying restlessness and producing sleep in nervous disorders. They should be moistened with water containing a trace of glycerin previously to being placed under the head of the patient in order to prevent rustling.

How to Make a Hop Pillow

To prepare your hop pillow, use a small muslin bag. Fill the bag loosely with dried hops and attach it to your regular pillow. The hops should be renewed every month.

Some people sprinkle a little alcohol on their hop pillows, claiming that it helps bring out the sedative properties of the plant.

CHAPTER SUMMARY

1. Calcium and pantothenic acid, also contained in selected herbs, have been found helpful in coping with insomnia and in curbing the distressing habit of tooth grinding during sleep.
2. Centuries of experience have confirmed that harmless specific herbs can be used to encourage sleep; they relieve tension, act as tranquilizers, and are non-habit forming.
3. Herbal sleep aids may be used in three ways:

- Herb teas
- Herbal baths
- Herbal scent-therapy (bedding scented with fragrant herbs; pillows stuffed with hops)

4. Herbal practitioners point out that since there are different causes of insomnia a specific herb tea may help one person and not another. By selecting one herb remedy at a time, and using it for four or five days, you will be able to find the formula best suited to your own personal need.

8

Legendary Occult Powers of Herbs

Is the holly or mistletoe part of your Christmas decorations? Do you throw rice at weddings? Knock on wood? Carry a four-leaf clover?

If your answer to any of these questions is "yes," then you, along with millions of others today, are still practicing the ancient art of plant-magic.

Superstition affects everyone from the most primitive to the most highly sophisticated. At times even hard core skeptics will grudgingly admit that superstition cannot always be shrugged off as utter nonsense.

In studying plant lore it can be seen that certain identical legends and traditions make their appearance in every part of the world and in many widely separated localities, forming as it were the basis of a vast universal system of folklore. This suggests that a great number of plant myths are founded mainly on fact rather than fancy. One illustration is plant symbology, the attempts by man to associate his more subtle emotions with the characteristics of certain plants or flowers. The spotless white lily could never represent anything but purity; the heliotrope, ever turning toward the sun, is a symbol of devotion; rosemary with its lingering color remains an eternal symbol of remembrance; the lofty palm is a widespread representation of victory; the olive branch has been throughout history a universal symbol of peace.

And it is a fact than many old and seemingly worthless herbal folk remedies have been proved by science to be of value after all.

As we look closely into the ancient mysteries of plant magic we shall find that the underlying principle upon which certain legends are based has become clouded but not lost.

OCCULT PLANT LORE

The Witches' Magic Salve

In every land and age we find legends of witches straddling their broomsticks while speeding along to the Sabbath through the heart of a dark raging tempest, their yells and hideous cackles sounding over the crash of elements. And we are told the flight was preceeded by anointing the body (generally the forehead and arm pits) with magic herbal salve.

The witch's broomstick was, of course, a symbol and not an incredible means of aerial transportation. Like the magician's wand, the shepherd's staff, or the Pharoah's scepter, it represented power and authority.

The magic salve, however, was an entirely different matter. It is thought to have first been introduced into Germany during the Middle Ages by roving bands of gypsies. Recipes given for the ointment included poisonous plants—henbane, deadly nightshade, and thorn apple. Witches claimed it was the salve or ointment that gave them power to fly through the air and in effect carried them to the Sabbath.

A Modern Test of the Witches' Salve

That the witches knew what they were talking about seems evident from experiments performed several years ago by a German professor, Dr. Will-Erich Peuckert, who decided to test the ancient formula. He followed the prescription carefully and concocted the salve with which he then anointed both himself and an attorney friend who knew nothing whatever about the effects the salve might produce. Both men immediately fell into a deep trance which lasted for 20 hours. With the return to consciousness they found their experiences during the trance state had been identical. Both told of the sensation of flying through the air, diving and plunging from dizzy heights, and of finally landing atop a mountain where they attended the celebration of the witches' Sabbath with its weird orgies and erotic activities. Dr. Peuckert concluded that the sorcerers of old did indeed celebrate the diabolical Sabbath although their experiences when using the ointment were not physical but psychic.

All this raises many questions. Why for instance does the salve produce exactly the same psychic effects in each person? Can an individual simply "dream" of something for which there was no precedent in mind? Does the salve perhaps stimulate a portion of racial memory? Or are such experiences simply hullucinations, as some psychologists maintain?

Other Vision-Producing Plants

Man has always used vision-producing plants in an attempt to break the barriers of sense limitation. In olden times this practice was thought to put one in touch with gods or devils; or enable one to discover hidden secrets, locate stolen or lost objects, divine the future; or give one the feeling of "being outside of one's self and transported to another world." This world could be hellish or heavenly, the vision beautiful or terrifying.

Because of their illuminating properties, such plants were held as sacred and used ceremoniously. It has long been known in primitive societies that a ritual setting is needed to channel the dangerous forces which a hallucinogenic drug releases. In other words the ritual helps the drug user to control the mind to a definite end, for example an oracular state of trance, rather than losing its sense of direction and being swept along by the force of the drug itself.

A few of the great many traditional plants used in primitive cultures include *ololiuqui,* the "devil's morning glory"; *Ayahuasca,* "soul vine" of the Amazon; *hashish,* the "god plant" of some Arab sects; *cohoba,* "magic snuff" of the Carribbean; and henbane, datura, and belladonna. Henbane gets its name from the fact that chickens often die from eating it.

The Magic Mushroom

Another secret plant used to send the mind to another world or into the future is the magic mushroom *(Amanita muscaria).*

Siberian medicine men or shamans drink broth from stewed *Amanita muscaria* for psychic experiences and for increased power of muscular strength and physical endurance. Travelers have reported seeing a drugged shaman dance continuously for hours, leaping as high as six feet into the air over and over again. According to Norse history, men who used a potion of the magic mushroom possessed uncanny strength and skill in battle. Because of their super physical power and their wild frenzy which no opponent could withstand, plus the fact that they fought clad only in a bearskin or "bersark," such men were called *berserk*—a word still used in our vocabulary today.

The Indians of Mexico and Central America call the sacred mushroom Teonanacatl,"flesh of the gods," and use it to produce visions, ecstasy and prophecy. Evidence indicates the Greeks also had knowledge of a similar species of mushroom which they called "food of the gods."

In addition to production of intense excitement, mushroom intoxication causes the shape and size of objects to appear distorted. Siberian explorers during the 18th and 19th centuries drew attention to these strange effects in their reports on the use of the sacred mushroom by Siberian peasants. It has been suggested that Lewis Carroll, author of *Alice in Wonderland,* used this information as a basis for a scene in his fairy tale where Alice is told by a caterpillar that if she wishes to grow large she should eat from one side of the toadstool and from the other side if she would grow small.

The psychic effects resulting from the use of the sacred mushroom are attributed to three highly dangerous alkaloids which the plant contains—muscarine, bufotenin, atropine. Muscarine is the constituent responsible for inducing pronounced physical power and endurance. However, directly following these marked effects, muscarine then acts as a poison paralyzing the nerves. Such paralysis is responsible for the deaths that often occur from accidental use of this mushroom.

The chemical bufotenin is also secreted from the sweat glands of the African toad (Bufo-bufotenesis), and it is curious to note that ancient legends associate certain toads with various species of mushrooms, claiming that both plants and animals are poisonous.

Yet it was only in recent years that science discovered bufotenin, a poison in the African and European toads. This drug is known to produce hallucinations in humans.

Peyote—the Divine Intoxicant of the Aztecs

Peyote (*Lophophora williamsii*), a small cactus with dried disk-like tips (mescal buttons), is of special interest because it is used today as a sacrament by the Native American Church, a religion based on Indian practices. The Article of Incorporation of this church reads that with the use of peyote worshippers are "able to absorb God's Spirit in the same way as the white Christian absorbs the Spirit by means of the sacramental bread and wine."

The Aztecs called the plant *peyotl* and ate the buttons ceremoniously either in the dried or green state. Peyote intoxication produces exhilaration followed by nausea, chills, and wakefulness, and finally brilliant color visions are seen, sometimes in geometric patterns which may shift and change into beautiful buildings or scenes stretching out into a limitless horizon. The kaleidoscopic play of colors is attributed to mescaline, an alkaloid contained in the mescal buttons. This property led the Indians to use the plant in religious ceremonies.

The standard peyote ritual among most Indian tribes still takes place in a tipi filled with the smell of sage, thyme, and burning logs. The ceremonial fire is situated between the horns of a crescent-shaped earthen mound.

During the all-night meeting, the leader prays to the peyote, beseeching its help and asking that it produces no ill effects on the users. Still directing his remarks to the plant, he promises to pray to it again at midnight and again in the morning. The number of peyote buttons eaten by each of the worshipers is generally four.

After certain purifying ceremonies have been completed, a carved staff, special drum and gourd rattle are passed around as each participant sings four peyote songs. Various water ceremonies occur at midnight and dawn when there is a baptismal rite followed by a special ritual breakfast.

The early Spanish missionaries protested against the use of peyote by the Indians and asked the penitent during the confessional: "Hast thou drunk *peyotl* or given it to others to drink, in order to discover secrets, or to discover where stolen or lost articles were?"

Dr. Francesco Hernandez, physician to the King of Spain, was also well-acquainted with the Indian use of Peyote. He wrote: "The *peyotl* causes those devouring it to be able to foresee and to predict things; such for instance, as whether the weather will continue favorable; or to discern who has stolen from them some utensil or anything else; and other things of like nature which the Chichimecas [a tribe of Mexican Indians] really believe they have found out."

The Mescalero ate peyote to detect rival witchcraft, find lost or stolen objects, and to foresee the future; the Osage and Oto used it in their funeral meetings to communicate with the dead. In Mexico the plant was employed for the purpose of prophesy or divination.

PSYCHIC PROTECTION THROUGH
THE POWER OF PLANT MAGIC

Today many people associate certain extraordinary occurrances of misfortune with what they call bad luck, chance, fate, or God's will. But in olden times such things were blamed on devils, evil spirits, witches, or sorcerers. All were malevolent, and their activities explained why a particular misfortune affected one person and not another at a precise moment in time. By cultivating a gentle or generous behavior, a wise individual could, at least to some extent, avoid the evils of witchcraft or sorcery. But if a man was spiteful, jealous, ill-tempered, or greedy, he risked the malice of his neighbors who might seek revenge through the services of a witch.

To cope with these evil forces people forearmed themselves with magic plants, especially before engaging in any activity or event which involved unpredictable risk, such as traveling, hunting, marriage, or business ventures. But should the evil strike before the victim managed to obtain the charmed plant, other herbs, roots, or barks were then used in an attempt to break the hex or spell.

How Plant Magic Works

Magic is not based on trickery but on the knowledge of natural laws which most people do not realize exist, or do not ordinarily know how to utilize for their personal benefit. Primitive man's magic dealt with all kinds of problems, and if the shaman or witch doctor didn't give some concrete evidence that they could do things no average individual could do, they would not have been looked upon with such awe and fear.

In recent years parapsychology has demonstrated that thought forces are electro-magnetic fields that cling to objects. In other words, everything we touch or handle becomes "charged" with our personal force field and this makes it possible for a good psychometrist to read our thoughts, character, and background, simply by holding in his hand any object belonging to us.

Primitive people knew about this power thousands of years ago and used it for magnetizing charms, amulets and talismans. A symbol, image, or object which has been deliberately charged with emotional thought-force can be a very effective link between the power it represents and the one who uses it.

How Charms Are Magnetized

When magnetizing a charm, amulet or talisman, the person holds the object in his hand and directly in front of his eyes. He then sets up concentrated emotional feelings of protection, wealth, love, or whatever the case may be, which he then directs like a power-beam toward the charm, visualizing his thoughts and emotions traveling from himself to the innermost depths of the object. As a result, the charm becomes charged with power somewhat like a battery storing up energy. These specially prepared objects gradually lose their power over a long period of time and have to be recharged.

Of course the effectiveness of any magnetized object is increased through the power of auto-suggestion—suggestion to the self of the idea associated with the charm. But it is necessary to point out definitely that favorable results are by no means due to suggestion alone.

It is also helpful if the shape and/or appearance of the object has some association with the magical purpose for which it is employed. In this way, every time the bearer looks at the charm a mental picture of its purpose is immediately triggered, and this keeps the mind steadily vibrating on a highly receptive and optimistic level.

A talisman, amulet, or charm works then if the three elements— emotional thought-force, conviction, shape and/or appearance—are properly combined. However, where plants are used in magic we shall see later on that in some instances other elements are involved, for the plant itself contains remarkable psychic properties.

THE OCCULT PLANTS

Let us take a few glimpses into the fascinating and curious world of plant myth and magic. You will notice here and there as we go along that the principle of shape and/or appearance is quite apparent with respect to charms, amulets, and talismans.

The Lucky Clover

Superstitions regarding the lucky clover have lingered in the minds of men almost longer than those of any other plant. The generic term *Trifolium* means one leaf with three parts, while the common name of clover is a corruption of the word Clava, a club. According to various legends it was placed on the playing cards because of its association with good luck. To many people the threefold leaf is an emblem of love, faith, and hope.

At night the clover undergoes a marked change, for as evening arrives the side leaves fold together and the center leaf bends over as though in prayerful adoration. This performance was undoubtedly an additional reason for the reverence in which the plant was held. It may also account for the idea which still prevails that it acts as a counter-charm against bad luck.

Occasionally a clover leaf is found that has four parts; this is widely accepted as a token of great fortune. One quaint country rhyme puts it this way:

> One leaf for fame,
> And one leaf for wealth
> And one for a faithful lover,
> And one to bring you glorious health
> Are all in a four-leaf clover.

St. John's Wort

From earliest times people have accepted as perfectly natural the idea that man has a body and a soul. At death the body was easily disposed of, but what to do with the soul or spirit was a different matter. Special rituals were developed and performed to "honor" the dead, but these were not so much reverence for the departed as fear of what the disembodied spirit could do to the living. In short, the ritual was really a way for people to protect themselves from the wrath of the dead. The problem of demons and uncanny beings who had never lived among mortals was also handled by special rituals.

Another way for one to protect one's self was the use of powerful plant-magic. In this category we find that St. John's Wort *(Hypericum perforatum)* ranks first. Its reddish colored sap represents the blood of St. John the Baptist, and the plant is consecrated to him. The generic name, *Hypericum*, clearly shows that the herb was highly regarded as having power over evil spirits. It is taken from two Greek words, *hyper* and *eikon* ("over" and "apparition"). In former times the herb was called *Fuga daemonum* or *Scare devil.*

To the early Christians the yellow stamens and bright golden flowers of St. John's Wort suggested the light of the sun, just as the Baptist was a "bright and shining light." This was "proof" of the herb's effectiveness as a safeguard against all forces of evil since the spirits of darkness hated the light; neither would they come to it, lest their deeds be reproved. Satan had no power over anyone who carried a talisman of St. John's Wort.

The plant was gathered on St. John's Day, June 24th, and hung over the door or window. In some lands it was burned in the Midsummer fires for various magical purposes, or worn as an amulet or charm.

Although St. John's Wort is still widely used today as an herbal remedy for wounds and certain illnesses, it was originally employed as a medicine for treating insanity, especially when the cause was thought to be demonic possession. Among some races it is still customary to burn the herb, the smoke and flame being considered especially potent for dispelling all types of evil influences.

Other Plants Consecrated to the Divine

St. John's Wort is by no means the only plant consecrated to a divine personage. The great white lily, for example, is one of the many floral emblems of the Madonna, the pure white petals representing her virginity, the golden anthers signifying her soul shining with divine light. Chamomile *(Matricaria)* is consecrated to St. Anne, mother of the Virgin. The botanical name, *Matricaria,* is from *mater* and *cara*—"beloved mother."

Plants called St. Christopher's Herb included the water fern, meadowsweet, life everlasting, and others. The water fern seems to be in reference to the legend of St. Christopher in which he is usually represented as wading through a river, bearing the Christ Child on his shoulders.

The oak was profoundly sacred to the Druids, and was also the tree under which Abraham was said to have received his heavenly visitors.

The Magic of the Yew and Holly

The powers of evil hated the yew and found the holly equally obnoxious, the reason being that the yew was generally found growing in churchyards and the word "holly" is similar in sound to the word "holy." To the early Christians, however, the thorny foliage and flaming red berries of the holly represented the crown of thorns with drops of blood falling to the ground. They claimed this to be the true reason the herb was magically protective when brought into the home, shielding mortals from evil spirits that wandered over the land during bleak winter months.

According to other legends, holly blessed the home with prosperity and good fortune provided the plant was not removed from the Christmas decorations until the New Year, and in some countries it was never disturbed until Candlemas Day (February 2).

Plants That Trap Evil Influences in the Home

The power to trap any type of evil influence which has been directed toward the home was attributed to onions and garlic! It is well known that the Chinese, Egyptians, Arabs, and other races still use them for this purpose. Either of the plants is selected and the bulb sliced, then suspended or set in the rooms of a house. The next morning the slices are carefully removed, burned, and replaced with fresh ones.

The onion was also credited with the power of protecting the home from contagion during epidemics and plagues. As recently as the 19th century many physicians still advocated placing sliced onions in the home as a preventive measure in such cases. Children wore onions in bags around their necks to ward off colds and other winter diseases.

Rue—the Occult Herb for the Psychic Faculties

Rue was used as a counter-charm against black magic. Legends indicating it was especially valued as an occult herb for awakening or sharpening the psychic faculties can be found the world over. For example, in the Tyrol people carried the herb in order to "sense the presence of witches."

Rue was so deeply revered in the British Isles that it was called the Herb of Grace, and missionaries sprinkled holy water with brushes made of it.

The Mystic Mandrake

Few plants have gathered such wealth of tradition and legend as that of a European herb known as mandrake. It should be carefully noted that the American species of mandrake *(Podophyllum peltatum)* is an entirely different variety although it bears the same common name. The ancient "magic" mandrake of Europe is a member of the deadly nightshade family and is known botanically as *Atropa mandragora.* The Romans believed it to be under the protection of Atropos, the grim-visaged Fate who mercilessly severed the thread of life which was spun by Clotho and the length of which was determined by Lachesis. The Greeks dedicated the plant to Circe, the golden-haired enchantress who was renowned for her knowledge of witchcraft.

Since the root is often forked, bearing a vague resemblance to the human form, mandrake was given the synonym of "earth-man" or "earth-mannikin." Many superstitions associated with the plant are due to this resemblance. The Romans called the herb *Semihomo*, while the Greeks referred to it as *Anthropomorphon*, both names indicating the human likeness. In Germany, mandrake was called the Sorcerer's Root, while the Arabs knew it as Satan's Apple or Devil's Apple.

Strange Medicinal Properties

Mandrake contains narcotic properties similar to those of belladonna. In early times the plant was used medicinally as an emetic (to cause vomiting). A potion called Morion or Death Wine was prepared from the roots and employed as an anesthetic for surgical operations. Mandrake was also cited as a rejuvenator as well as a cure for sterile women, and it is still used for the latter purpose today in Africa and the Far East. Recently, Indian scientists in Bombay, studying the physiological activity of plants, have reported that sterile women given an extract prepared from European mandrake have consistently given birth to boy babies!

Mandrake's Dramatic Reputation

Many of the legends concerning mandrake are intensely dramatic, and sometimes gruesome. It was said the herb grew only in dark foreboding places or under the shadow of the gallows "nourished by the exhalations from executed criminals." Another curious tale claims the plant clung so desperately to the ground that when uprooted it screamed like a tormented human, and its cries brought madness or instant death to anyone hearing them. To avoid these dangerous or lethal effects, the harvester plugged his ears with beeswax, then tied a dog to the herb. The animal was then called or enticed away. As the root was torn from the earth its heart-rending shrieks caused the unfortunate dog to drop dead on the spot!

Power for Good or Evil

Fascinating tales of the magic and marvels connected with possession of the mandrake root were rife. It was worn as an amulet, employed as an oracle, and treasured as a potent substance in all forms of magical arts. A letter written in 1675 by a burgomaster of Leipzig is extant which clearly demonstrates the superstitions that prevailed in those times regarding the occult use of this herb. The burgomaster had heard that his brother was suffering from a series of great misfortunes, so he purchased a mandrake root and sent it to him with the following instructions:

> When thou hast the Earth-Man in thy house, let it rest for three days without approaching it; then place it in warm water. With the water afterwards sprinkle the animals, the sills of the house, going over all, and soon it shall all go better with thee, and thou shalt come to thy own if thou serve the Earth-Mannikin right. Bathe it four times every year, and as often wrap it in silk cloths and lay it among thy best things and thou need do no more. The bath in which it hath been bathed is especially good. When thou goest to law, put the mannikin under thy right arm, and thou shalt succeed, whether right or wrong.

Note the total conviction expressed in this letter that the charm will work. Bathing the herb, wrapping it in silk cloths, etc., are rudimentary forms of magnetizing.

Earlier beliefs in which mandrake was associated with the devil continued almost until modern times. Madame du Noyer cited an incident in which the murder of Marechal de Fabert was popularly attributed to a broken contract with the devil. Later, two mandrakes of remarkable beauty were found in his room, and these were considered by his friends as evidence of his pact with Satan.

HERBS AND THE EVIL EYE

Since the eyes convey love or hatred, peace or agression, joy or sorrow, it appeared likely that an evil mind was projected through the eyes—hence the "evil eye."

To those who believed in this power a mere glance was enough to cause a variety of misfortunes, but it was generally agreed that particularly penetrating eyes were the ones to be shunned at all costs. Fascinated, bewitched, enchanted—these were some of the words used to describe the effects of this type of diabolical activity.

In ancient times, belief in the evil eye was so widespread that Greek philosophers tried to find an explanation for the enigma and came up with the idea that the eyes emitted powerful rays which could strike external objects. But it was only a few years ago that modern science began entertaining similar thoughts. When the subject of Human Radiations was discussed at a meeting held in New York by the American Association for the Advancement of Science, Professor Otto Kahn reported that the power of the human eye could kill yeast cells used in making bread! A glass in which the yeast cells were placed was held close to the subject's eye. Staring through the glass at the cells for only a few minutes brought about their death. Professor Kahn was quick to add, however, that human radiations have also been found to be highly beneficial.

Legendary Methods for Diverting the Evil Eye

In olden times many different forms of plant magic were used as a protection against the evil eye. Some plants allegedly diverted fascination by their odor, others by their color, and still others by their strange performance or some peculiarity of shape. Frankincense, myrrh, sandalwood, or other fragrant botanicals were burned or strewn around the home.

To bathe the eyes with water in which the herb rue had been steeped was another popular method for preventing or breaking the spell. The power of bestowing second sight (clairvoyant vision) was also attributed to this "magic water," and Milton, the famous English poet, depicts Michael as purging Adam's eyes with it:

> To nobler sights
> Michael from Adam's eyes the film removed
> Which that false fruit which promized clearer sight
> Had bred; then purged with Euphrasie and Rue
> The visual nerve, for he had much to see.

Evil Eye in Modern Times

That the long tradition of the evil eye is still with us is evident in our modern speech when we speak of a dirty look, an icy stare, a piercing glance, or a whammy. It is also apparent from the numerous incidents that are continually being reported whereby misfortune is attributed to "fascination." For example, an English publication, *The Countryman,* stated that the older people in Somerset believed the evil eye had caused cattle to die, and a pig to go berserk. And several years ago an incident in which the evil eye was allegedly used to keep dissatisfied workers on the job was brought to the attention of the U.S. Senate labor rackets investigating committee. According to news reports the committee's lawyer said: "He was hired by one employer to come in once or twice every week or so and glare at his employees." This, it seemed, was enough "to keep them at work."

MISCELLANEOUS OCCULT
AND MYSTIC USES OF HERBS

The Magic Wand

The belief that rods prepared from the branches of certain trees can be used to reveal hidden underground water or metals dates from antiquity. Among the ancient Greeks we find this type of "magic" under the term *rhabdomancy,* "divination by means of a rod." In olden times the rod was often called the magic wand or wishing rod. Engravings 4000 years old show Emperor Yu of China using a divining rod.

The Chinese prefer to cut their rods from fruit trees such as the peach. Others employ rowan, osier, or blackthorn, but witch hazel has always been the favorite. The word "witch" in this case refers to the pliability of the wood, and comes from the Anglo-Saxon *wic-en,* "to bend." The rod is shaped somewhat like the letter Y and is held by the forked parts, allowing the tip or end to point outward.

Methods for procuring and preparing the rod were numerous. For example: "In cutting it, one must face the east, so that the rod shall be one which catches the first rays of the morning sun, or as some say, the eastern and western sun must shine through the

fork of the rod, otherwise it will be good for nothing." An
identical legend prevails in China regarding the rod cut from the
peach tree, and even in the time of the Vedas similar instructions
were given to the Hindus for cutting the *cami* branch and the
arani.

Toward the end of the 17th century Vallemont wrote an
extensive treatise on the use of the divining rod or *baguette
divinatoire.* In it he gives the story of a "countryman who, guided
by his rod, pursued a murderer by land for a distance exceeding
forty-five leagues, besides thirty leagues more by water."

The divining rod is still known and used the world over, not
only in searching for hidden water, but also for locating oil, lost
mines, buried treasure and even missing persons. Modern business
firms have been known to hire skilled dowsers to help discover oil
or underground streams, and in many cases the dowsers have
proved highly successful.

Plant Indicators

According to folk lore there is another way in which the plant
world can be helpful in locating valuable minerals or precious ores
hidden in the earth. Wild buckwheat *(Eriogonum ovalifolium)*,
native to the western parts of the United States, is said to thrive in
abundance where silver may be found; locoweed often reveals
uranium deposits; copper is indicated when the California poppy is
found growing in Arizona; the tumbleweed and a plant known as
milk vetch are said to grow in areas of selenium deposits. In
England it is claimed that coal is hidden deeply underground
wherever the herb coltsfoot grows. In Germany, coltsfoot is
believed to indicate deposits of lead.

The notion that certain plants are indicators of valuable ore
deposits is rapidly gaining support in some scientific circles.
Reports coming from Venezuela state that a variety of copei tree
which thrives only on soil produced by iron ore has a specific
texture on aerial photographs which can lead engineers and
scientists to underground ore deposits from photographs of the
area. Scientific researchers in other countries are also taking a keen
interest in plants as indicators of hidden ores.

Strange Mystic Attachments of Herbs and Plants

In many countries it is believed that strange mystic attachments exist between certain plants and other forms of life. Persian legends claim the nightingale utters a plaintive cry whenever a rose is plucked. In the springtime the bird allegedly hovers around the flower until overcome by its fragrance. You may place a handful of scented herbs and flowers before the nightingale, but he will spurn them all and remain constant and faithful to his beloved rose.

The legend that sage will thrive or decline as the master's business prospers or fails is still widespread. Accounts of the strange rapport of plants with the trials and successes of individuals have been recorded. In Friend's *Flowers and Flower Lore* we find the following:

> It is said that one of the great treasures in the Hohenzollern Museum at Berlin is a fragment of wood from an ancient pear tree at the foot of the Unsterberg, near Salzburg, which, according to tradition, would blossom and bear so long as the German Empire flourished, but would die with the fall of the Imperial power. In 1806, when the Empire was dissolved, and the Confederation of the Rhine formed, the tree withered away, and the poet Chamisso alluded to the old legend in one of his poems. The tree remained lifeless for over sixty years, but in 1871, after the establishment of the new German Empire, the old trunk suddenly put forth branches, blossomed, and bore fruit.

MODERN SCIENCE REVEALS
HIDDEN PSYCHIC NATURE OF PLANTS

We have just covered a few of the great many legends pertaining to the magical power of trees, herbs, roots, and flowers. And now that you have become familiar with them, let us acquaint ourselves with the work of modern researchers who have discovered some amazing facts about the hidden psychic nature of plants. We shall see that their findings relate, in a remarkable and almost unbelievable way, to some of the legends we have just considered.

Scientist Discovers Plant ESP

Cleve Backster was Chairman of the Research Committee of the Academy for Scientific Interrogation for eight years and has designed some of the polygraph (lie detector) equipment used today. A polygraph is employed for testing a subject's emotional reactions, and best results are achieved when the subject is made to feel that his well-being is threatened. To determine if plants could experience emotions, Backster wired up a green leafy subject, and then tried to think of something drastic he could do that would pose a threat to its life. The thought occurred that he might burn the plant. At that precise moment the needle on the chart shot upward. Backster was astonished, for the record on the chart indicated the plant had just read his mind!

For more than three years Backster continued experimenting with plants, repeating many different tests over and over, always obtaining the same remarkable results. Then in 1959 his first report on his findings was published in the *International Journal of Parapsychology*. Today, the polygraph expert is still conducting his plant experiments. So far his findings seem to indicate that plants have intelligence, emotions, memories, and an ESP communicative process capable of reaching great distances instantaneously! Several universities across the country are now repeating some of his experiments.

Here are a few examples of the remarkable effects Backster obtained with plants:

Three plants with electrodes attached were placed in separate office rooms. A specially constructed machine located at the far end of the hall was geared to automatically dump live brine shrimp into boiling water at random times. Backster threw the switch on the machine, then left the office. The next morning when he returned he found that each of the plants had registered an emotional reaction at the precise moment of the shrimp's death.

In another experiment, one of six men was chosen by lot to "murder" a plant. Each of the men entered a room in which two plants had been placed. When the last man had filed out, Backster went into the room and found one of the plants torn to pieces. He attached his instruments to the survivor, a philodendron, and asked the six men to re-enter the room one by one. The moment the "killer" appeared the philodendron showed an immediate emotional reaction!

One of Backster's most interesting findings was that plants have more love for human beings than for any other form of life. Although their reaction to the extinction of other life forms loses intensity after the experiments have been repeated over and over, they never seem to get used to the death of human cells (a wound cleansed with antiseptic, for example).

But that is not all. Plants apparently know if you really love them or not, and seem quite capable of establishing emotional relationships with humans. Backster, who treats his plants with tender care, has found that if he becomes upset about anything, even though he may be blocks away from his office at the time, his plants react. Their greatest emotional response is registered when he is actually on his way back to the office.

Every plant apparently has this close affection for its owner. Backster recalls the time a friend left a house plant with him while she was vacationing out of town. He attached the electrodes and found the plant registered an emotional response the very moment its owner's plane landed in another state! It seems the plant reflected the woman's nervousness and stress during the landing operation.

Plants and Herbs Are Like People

Over 50 years ago, some equally remarkable experiments were conducted in Calcutta, India, by the late Sir Jaghadish. Using highly sensative and delicate instruments he was able to measure a plant's movements associated with shock, growth, and response to stimuli in general. Results obtained from these and thousands of other tests led Sir Jaghadish to draw the following conclusions:

Plants not only have consciousness, they also have their moods, their whims, their good days and bad. A plant struck a violent blow shakes and quivers in veritable agony. A plant yanked up by the roots experiences a shock comparable to that of a person beaten into insensibility. Each plant has a marked personality, along with racial and family traits.

Plants exhibit the same hopes, the same logic, and undergo the same trials as man, but in a lesser degree.

As every gardener knows, many trees and plants fail to survive transplanting and die of shock even if their tissues are not injured in any way. Sir Jaghadish performed an interesting experiment in which he administered a chemical that acted as an anesthetic to trees about to be transplanted. He found they stood the relocation very well but some cases showed an apparent loss of memory and a general state of upset, exactly as a man or animal would when coming out of a stupor.

Plant Response to Prayer, Love, and Music

In recent years serious investigators have repeatedly demonstrated that plants will grow better and be healthier when prayed over. In other words, you can pray daily that your potted plant, shrubs, trees, or flowers will grow luxuriously. You can speak to them in a kindly way, saying for example: "I love you, please grow strong and healthy," and they will respond to the energy supplied by your prayers and expressions of love.

Music also has a decided effect on plant growth. Plants subjected to heavy doses (three hours daily) of rock 'n' roll for ten days leaned away from the loud speaker, began to wilt and shrivel, then finally collapsed and died. By contrast, those treated to classical, semi-classical, or soft melodious strains produced healthy foliage and beautiful blossoms, and grew taller than plants subjected to nothing but silence.

A MODERN SLANT ON THE OLD LEGENDS OF HERBS

Now let us take a second look at a few of the ancient legends about plant magic mentioned earlier in this chapter and see how they relate to the scientific findings we have just considered.

Legend of the Screaming Mandrake

Tests conducted by Sir Jaghadish showed that a plant pulled up by the roots suffers tremendous shock, comparable to that of a person beaten into insensibility. This immediately calls to mind the legend of the screaming mandrake. Perhaps the myth originated when some person here and there with mediumistic ability tore a mandrake from the ground and psychically sensed the plant's torment and anguish. Such an experience would have excited profound emotions of horror in the mind of the psychic, especially if the person was a timid soul or one whose psychic faculties had just emerged for the first time. It is not difficult to understand that in some instances the shock could have caused insanity or heart failure.

How the Power of the Onion and Garlic Works

Psychic researchers maintain that intense emotional energy can become impressed upon the atmosphere of a room, house, or locality just as the impressions of sound can be received by a tape recorder. Although these forces are invisible they are there. If a sensitive person should enter an emotionally charged area his mind absorbs the lingering thought-forces, and he experiences a sense of foreboding, gloom, anxiety, stress, or any other type of mental state, depending on the quality and nature of the emotion he is contacting.

To some researchers this theory also accounts for certain types of hauntings in which a ghost or apparition is repeatedly seen in the same room or area and always acting in exactly the same way. In cases of this kind the emotional energy resulting from some act, suicide or murder for example, becomes impressed on the atmosphere of a room like an image locked into a photographic emulsion. In other words, the "ghost" is not actually there, but what is seen is a sort of photographic replay of a tragedy that occurred sometime in the past.

Now you will note that the legend of garlic and onions refers specifically to their power of trapping "evil influences" *in the home.* If we accept the theory of an emotionally charged atmosphere, and the evidence that plants have intelligence, ESP, and the ability to react whenever their well-being is threatened, the ancient legend deserves serious consideration. Assuming the theory is valid, if garlic and onions are placed in "haunted" rooms or houses they could become psychically aware of the dangerous emotional particles clinging to the atmosphere, and might react by trapping and destroying them.

A possible clue to their lethal effects on "psychic germs" may lie in the discoveries of Professor Alexander Gurwitch, a Russian electro-biologist who found that garlic and onions emit a strange type of ultraviolet radiation which he called M-rays. These mysterious rays may also account for the persistent legendary claims that the humble onion protects the home from contagion. Another factor which may provide a clue here is the ethereal oil which both the garlic and the onion contain, and which is responsible for their strong penetrating odor and hot blistering effects.

Success of Peyote Ritual Revealed

It is well known that people who have tried peyote independently have not obtained the same noteworthy effects in the form of spiritual revelations, ecstasy, or clairvoyance that the Indian experiences through his peyote ritual. And it is important to note that scientific testimony over the past 50 years has shown that peyote *as used ceremoniously by the Indians* never caused serious harm either morally, physically, or psychically.

The necessity for a ceremony when using powerful hallucinogenic plant drugs has already been pointed out, but two factors in the peyote ritual are of special interest: (1) During the all-night meeting the Indian leader prays over or talks directly to the peyote. (2) Each participant sings peyote songs. Here we have the combined elements of prayer and music which produce definite effects upon plants.

Plant Consecration

A plant, tree, or flower consecrated to a Divine personage would in effect become the property of the Holy being; and we have learned that plants have a strong attachment for their owners. Under the circumstances it is possible that by means of ESP a plant, such as St. John's Wort for example, could pierce the barrier between the here and the hereafter and form a relationship or bond with the departed saint. If so, the herb might become a sort of focal point for bringing a special blessing into the home of the individual, or to the individual himself who keeps the plant in his care. (Note the legend that heavenly hosts visited Abraham under a sacred oak.)

If a trance medium can slip in and out of both the physical and the spiritual worlds with ease, why not a consecrated psychic plant?

Strange Mystic Attachments Explained

In the light of the Backster experiments, the legends about sage, thriving or wilting as its owner's business prospers or fails, and about the negative or positive reaction displayed by the pear tree in direct correspondence with the rise and fall of the German Empire, are true. You will recall that Backster's pet plants showed a reaction whenever he became upset, and that his friend's house plant reflected its owner's apprehension when her plane landed.

Why these legends specifically mention sage and the pear tree seems a little puzzling as Backster's findings indicate that *all* plants have a strong attachment for their owners. However, it may be that some trees, herbs, or flowers are more emotionally sensitive than others.

What of the Nightingale and the Rose?

If plants have an attachment for all forms of life, it is not unreasonable to assume that in some cases the reverse could also be true. If so, it is quite possible the nightingale senses the traumatic shock the rose experiences when plucked.

The Magic Wand

Many theories have been advanced regarding the power of the divining rod to make some movement just as the operator or dowser passes over an area of land that contains the underground stream of water or hidden treasure. The most popular concept is that the subconscious mind always reaches out to obtain the desired information, but the impressions received back by the conscious mind are so vague or subtle that the divining rod is needed as a sort of amplifier to make the impressions clear cut to the dowser.

We would like to suggest another possibility. If plants possess ESP along with a strong attachment for their owners, perhaps the divining rod senses the desire of its master and guides him by means of ESP.

And the traditional instructions given for cutting the rod may have some deep significance. Perhaps the sun's rays "recharge" the life force or electromagnetic field of the severed branch, enabling the rod to retain its particles of psychic energy. Belief on the part of the operator that the rod cut in this fashion will work is an added factor.

We realize of course that many modern dowsers use rods made of metal, in which case other theories are applied to account for their effectiveness. But in suggesting the theory just cited, we are speaking of rods made from branches.

CHAPTER SUMMARY

Occult herbs have always been held in great favor and it has only been possible to touch upon a few of the more popular in this survey.

Perhaps the most important fact that emerges is the poverty of our overall knowledge regarding the strange psychic principles in plants and within the human mind itself. But as our scientific world of the 20th century continues to take a greater interest in these mysteries we shall learn much more about our own hidden nature and that of our lesser brothers of the plant kingdom.

As of now, the following facts have been established:

1. Suggestion affects everyone, from the most primitive people to the most highly sophisticated.
2. From man's most distant past right up to the present day, release from the physical world and entry into the psychic and spiritual has been sought through vision-producing plants.
3. Primitives have always known that the framework of a magico-religious ritual is helpful for controlling the dangerous forces which a hallucinogenic plant drug releases.
4. An amulet, talisman, or plant charm works provided the elements of shape and/or appearance, magnetization, and conviction (belief that the charm will work) are properly combined.

5. Modern studies indicate that plants have intelligence, emotions, ESP, and the ability to form relationships with humans.
6. Music and prayer produce definite effects upon plants.
7. In the light of controlled scientific research we have at last been given a sound basis for understanding how the age-old plant myths and legends might have originated and perpetuated themselves.

9

Herbal Preparations for the Relief of Headaches and Tensions

Nature offers a generous supply of harmless but efficient herbs which can provide solace and help for persons troubled with stress, anxiety tension, or nagging headache pains. T. Bartram, a modern practitioner of natural therapeutics, says: "Valerian is still available for those who wish to explore safer roads back to a healthy nervous system. We plead for a return to plant medicine as old as time, in the place of modern drugs of questionable safety."

Valerian is an ancient herbal nervine and sedative. In 1951 Gstirner and Kind showed that its age-old reputation was a valid one. These two scientists discovered that the herb's calming effects were due to the cooperation of several of the plant's active ingredients.

TRANQUILITY WITHOUT DRUGS

Here is a brief list of some of the herbs that are employed as nervines in botanic medicine. (A number of other plants which may be used for their charming influence are cited in the chapter on insomnia.)

LADY'S SLIPPER *(Cypripedium pubescens)*

Synonyms: Nerve root, yellow moccasin, American valerian.
Part Used: The root.

The Penobscot and other Indian tribes boiled the root of lady's slipper herb and used the decoction as a nerve medicine. The remedy passed from the hands of the Indians to the early colonists and eventually found its way into the medical profession. In 1849 Dr. Porcher wrote that it was highly esteemed as an antispasmodic and sedative, its action being similar to valerian in alleviating nervous symptoms. It was reputed to be effective in the treatment of hysterical conditions and in chorea (a nervous disorder characterized by spasmodic twitchings and other involuntary movements).

Recorded Uses

Here is the medical opinion of Dr. Swinburne Clymer, M.D., on the value and use of lady's slipper:

"Lady's slipper powder is the best of known nervines. It will produce the most beneficial effects in all cases of nervous affections as also in hysterical symptoms. It is perfectly harmless, and may be used in all cases with safety, and is much better than the dangerous and habit-forming narcotics which number their victims by the millions. This powder has a tendency to promote sleep and is highly soothing, but this is due to its potency to quiet the nerves and to create a state of ease, permitting sleep during which nature may tone up the system and heal the afflictions. Half a teaspoonful may be given in hot water and the dose repeated as often as necessary."

MOTHERWORT *(Leonurus cardiaca)*

Synonyms: Lion's Tail, Lion's Ear.
Part Used: Herb.

That motherwort was employed centuries ago as a medicinal plant is indicated by the old English term "wort," while the prefix "mother" suggests its use in female disorders. Early herbalists claimed the herb had a beneficial effect on the womb and uterine membranes, and that it was also a specific remedy for nervous irritability and hysterical complaints. The botanical name *cardiaca* links the plant with the heart, and we find that motherwort was administered as a simple heart tonic, especially for palpitations.

Early claims for the herb's therapeutic action as a nervine and heart tonic are quite remarkable when we realize that the old herb doctors could not possibly have known that the plant contains an abundance of calcium. Scientists have found that this precious mineral is necessary for the health of the muscles. Since the heart is a muscle it requires calcium for strength and to regulate the rhythm of the heart beat. The body also requires calcium for controlling the electric impulses that are transmitted through the nerves.

Szekely writes: "Calcium is the dominant nerve controller and powerfully affects the cell formation of all living things and regulates nerve action. It governs contractability of muscles and rhythmic beat of the heart."

Motherwort has retained its age-old classification as tonic, nervine, antispasmodic, and emmenagogue, and is used much the same today as it was in the past. In addition to calcium, the plant also contains alkaloids, bitter principles, and a volatile oil.

Motherwort to the Rescue

"My patient had delivered a veritable 'organ recital.' " Dr. Jon Evans wrote. "Everything, it would appear, seemed to be wrong. The slightest thing caused her to be upset, often with heart palpitations; she was nervous and irritable and sometimes became hysterical when faced with an unusual degree of domestic pressure. Menstruation was irregular and difficult and just before the beginning of the cycle things appeared to be at their worst.

"Six months before our interview the patient had suffered from a severe attack of flu which had left her very weak and depressed; the palpitations had from that time increased, usually coinciding with some personal tension. A further symptom was a febrile condition at night. After taking the case history and making the appropriate examination, a medicine was prescribed prepared from the herb motherwort. It not only fitted the clinical picture, but it worked like a charm. In a short time the lady who had previously found life to be an 'endurance test' with a galaxy of unpleasant symptoms, became relaxed and calm; the wretched conditions which had plagued her for so long disappeared. It is interesting to note that the medicine consisted of a single herb, its action was effective and safe, and certainly it produced no side effects.

"As to preparation, an infusion can be made from the herb. One ounce to one pint of boiling water, to be taken in wineglassful doses three times a day after meals. . . . If the preparation is taken in the form of fluid extract the dose is ½ to 1 drachm."

SCULLCAP *(Scutellaria laterifolia)*

Synonyms: Quaker Bonnet, Hoodwort.
Part Used: Leaves, twigs.

The natural habitat of this plant is North America, Europe, and the eastern parts of Asia. The American species ranks first in medicinal value and quality.

Scullcap contains a volatile oil, fat, sugars, tannin, cellulose, mucilage, a bitter principle, a glycoside $C_{10}H_8O_2$ called *scutellarin*. The herb is said to act beneficially on the nervous system.

Recorded Uses

1. Scullcap. Tonic, nervine, antispasmodic, slightly astringent. Is one of the finest nervines ever discovered, and may be prescribed wherever disorders of the nervous system exist. . . . The dose, of an infusion of one ounce to one pint of boiling water, is half a teacupful frequently.[1]

2. *Scutellaria,* by its action through the cerebro-spinal centers, is a most valuable remedy, controlling nervous irritation, calming hysterical excitement. . . . In restlessness and excitement, with insomnia, following prolonged application to business, long sickness or physical exhaustion, it is most useful. When given in hot drinks it acts more quickly, and also brings on diaphoresis [sweating]. In treating heavy drinkers who wish to give up the habit, I know of nothing better than *Scutellaria.* It steadies and sobers the patient, and brings on sleep and appetite. *—Dr. Fearn—Lloyd's.*

3. Scullcap is one of the most reliable tonic nervines and best used in the form of an infusion from the herb, or the tincture in hot water.

In irritable, nervous conditions, *Scutellaria* should be combined with:

Tincture Cypripedium ½ oz.
Tincture Scutellaria 1 oz.

Dose 10 to 30 drops every 2 to 4 hours in water.[2]

---

[1] R.C. Wren, *Potter's New Cyclopedia of Botanical Drugs and Preparations,* (Sir Isaac Pitman & Sons Ltd., London) 7th ed. 1956.

[2] *Nature's Healing Agents,* (Quakertown, Pa: The Humanitarian Society, Reg.), 1960.

4. Nervous debility:

Fluid Extract Scullcap . . . . 3 drachms
Fluid Extract Valerian . . . . 3 drachms
Fluid Extract Mistletoe *(Viscum album)* . 3 drachms
Fluid Extract Hops . . . . 3 drachms
Fluid Extract Gentian . . . . 3 drachms

Add water to 8 ounces. Take two teaspoonfuls in water before meals.—*Medical Herbalist.*

Dr. J. R. Yemm gives this interesting account:

"A gentleman I met recently who appeared to be in robust health, informed me that for three years he had been continually under the treatment of various doctors for nervous debility and insomnia. Treatment which included bromides and other drugs had been of no avail. Being induced to try natural medicine he prepared an infusion from scullcap, one ounce; hops, half-ounce; gentian root, crushed, half-ounce. After only one week of the herbal treatment he was sleeping well; at the end of two months fully recovered."

VALERIAN *(Valeriana officinalis)*

Synonyms: All Heal, Setwall, English Valerian.
Part Used: Root

Valerian is a perennial herb native to Europe and Asia. It is not to be confused with lady's slipper which is often called American valerian, although both herbs are said to produce similar therapeutic action.

Some authorities say that the name valerian is from the Latin *valere,* "to be in health," while others believe it takes its name from an ancient physician, Valerius, who was first to employ the herb in medicine. In early times the plant was so highly esteemed for its healing virtues that it was called "Blessed Herb" and dedicated to the Virgin Mary.

Valerian is a traditional remedy for functional disturbances of the nervous system, and was listed among the home-remedies in the domestic books of the 11th century. A remedy of the 15th century states: "Men who begin to fight and when you wish to stop them give the juice of Amantilla, *id est Valeriana* [valerian] and peace will be made immediately." In an article in the *British Medical Journal* published in 1928, Dr. Manson wrote that valerian "was perhaps the earliest method of treating the neurosis."

Today, valerian is employed by many orthodox physicians; unfortunately however it is generally combined with bromides, thus turning a valuable organic remedy into an inorganic one. Medical herbalists deplore the practice and prefer to use the herb alone, or in combination with other appropriate botanicals.

Constituents of Valerian

Valerian contains valerianic, formic and acetic acids, in addition to an essential oil, resin, starch, a glucoside, and two alkaloids—*chatrine* and *valerianine.* In botanic medicine the action of the root is classified as nervine, antispasmodic, sedative, anodyne, and carminative.

Recorded Uses

1. Dr. William Fox gives the following information on the medicinal value of valerian:

"It is especially useful in cases of nervous derangement, especially for nervous females, in hysterical, restless, and irritable conditions. Dose—of an infusion of the root, one or two wineglassfuls; of the tincture, 20 to 30 drops in sweetened water three or four times a day."

2. Dr. Clymer offers this suggestion: "In all extreme nervous conditions where the stomach is at fault, the best results will be obtained by giving the following combination:

> Tincture *Anthemis* [chamomile] 1 oz.
> Tincture valerian ¼ oz.

"Five to 30 drops every three hours or less, according to the severity of the symptons. . . ."

3. In reference to valerian, Dr. Yemm wrote:

"It is soothing and diffusive, gives relief in irritability of the nervous system, insomnia and hysteria, and is especially suitable to children's nervousness. It exerts a marked influence on the cerebro-spinal system, acting directly on those parts, thereby causing steadiness in unbalanced conditions. The root eases pain and promotes sleep. Those suffering from overstrained nerves find it especially beneficial.

"Preparation and uses—make the infusion as follows: Valerian, one ounce; water (boiling), one pint. Dose: one or two wineglassfuls four times daily."

4. Herbalists often combine valerian with two or more suitable plants. Here is a popular formula for nervous tension and restlessness. Mix:

> 1 tablespoon valerian
> 1 tablespoon scullcap
> 1 tablespoon catnip
> 1 teaspoon celery seeds

Prepare as an infusion with one pint of boiling water. Cover and allow to steep for ten minutes. Strain. The recommended dose is one cup of the hot tea three or four times a day. The beverage is sipped slowly.

WOOD BETONY *(Betonica officinalis)*

Synonyms: Bishopswort, Betony.
Part Used: Herb

The common name of this plant is derived from the Celtic *ben* (the head) and *ton* (good) in reference to its alleged virtues as a remedy for treating head complaints.

Antonius Musa, physician to Augustus Caesar, wrote a whole book on the remedial use of wood betony, and every herbalist century after century has praised the herb as a valuable plant medicine. An early herbarium written by Apuleius declares betony to be "good whether for man's soul or for his body; it shields him against frightful visions and dreams, and the wort is very wholesome." Turner in his *British Physician* 1687, said: "It would seem a miracle to tell what experience I have had with it, not only in cases of insomnia but in removing pain from any part of the head."

Recorded Uses

Wood betony is classified as nervine, sedative, tonic, alterative, astringent, and aromatic.

Dr. Jon Evans presents a good example of the way the herb is employed in modern times: "In medical practice I have found many patients suffering from nervous tension who get irritable and excited and complain of head pains of a purely functional nature. They also sleep badly, sometimes complaining of dreams. For this symptomatic picture I strongly commend wood betony. A simple infusion can be made with one ounce of the herb to one pint of boiling water. A wineglassful to be taken frequently."

NATURE'S HERBAL REMEDIES FOR COPING WITH HEADACHES

Migraine

An estimated 12 million Americans periodically suffer attacks of migrane headache. Scientists use the term "dols" as a measurement of pain. On a chart, six dols is given as the degree of pain the average person seldom exceeds. Intense migraine headache is listed at nine!

If the migraine victim is fortunate, the headache lasts under an hour; if he is not, it may last all day, and sometimes for several consecutive days, or even a week.

Symptoms of Migraine

The migraine sufferer is well acquainted with the various signs of an impending attack. Just prior to reaching the point of pain, the vision is affected in some way. Things begin to look hazy, misty, or blurry. Black spots or bright flashes of light may appear before the eyes. The victim may also feel dizzy. Shortly following these symptoms, a pounding, throbbing sensation of pain strikes one side of the head, generally over the right eye, but some people experience it over the left. In a matter of moments the pain reaches its full fury. In some cases it may eventually extend to the entire crown of the head and become a steady excruciating pain. And to compound the agony, an attack of migraine is almost always accompanied by nausea and vomiting.

Until the migraine is over, working or social activity is completely out of the question. Most victims can only suffer, lying quietly in a darkened room free from noise, until the attack wears itself out.

Some Possible Causes of Migraine

Here are some of the possible causes of migraine headache according to various medical opinions: (1) Low blood sugar, a condition which is usually the result of a diet rich in sugar and refined starches, and short in vitamins and minerals. (2) Forms of mental tension, such as grief, rage, shattering disappointments, and anxiety. (3) Liver trouble. (4) Constipation with resulting "auto-intoxication." (5) Allergy to preservatives and to chemical additives in food. (6) Glandular deficiencies, a conclusion which has been drawn from the fact that quite often migraine attacks cease in middle age when gland functions slow down (with men when they reach their 50's and with women at the time of menopause).

Wrong eating habits have also been found to trigger migraine. Dr. Atkinson says: "Perhaps the two most common faults are inadequate breakfast and an excess, often a gross excess, of carbohydrates. Diets should be high protein, low fat, medium carbohydrate, and consideration should be paid to the possibility of allergenic foods such as chocolate and cheese as etiological factors in migraine. Tobacco in Meniere's and alcohol in migraine should be limited or preferably prohibited, as being frequent and potent causes of trouble."

Although not many migraine victims realize it, inhalants and even certain odors can start the cycle that results in throbbing, blinding headaches. Dr. Spear tells us that house dust and mold are the most common among the offending inhalants. Patients allergic to house dust and mold may notice symptoms of headache after exposure to musty basements or after housecleaning. Dr. Spear says that the odors which may bring on a migraine attack are smog, paint, paint thinner, tobacco smoke, aerosols, perfumes, ammonia, chlorine, frying odors, motor exhaust, and formalde-hyde (a chemical used in some of the stay-press garments).

Vitamin Therapy

Note that vitamins are contained in herbs also.

Injections of a combination of vitamins B_1 and B_2 in high doses were reported by M. Atkinson *(The Practitioner,* 1958), as remarkably effective in cases of migraine headache. Another physician, Dr. Nevil Lyton, employs a combination which includes

B vitamin riboflavin, pyridoxine and nicotinamide, plus 800 milligrams of vitamin C in each injection. Sometimes Dr. Lyton uses riboflavin only in milder cases of migraine. Although he gives this vitamin by injection he says many other authorities report that ten milligrams three times a day taken orally has proved helpful.

Relief from Migraine Through Vitamin C

One man found complete relief from migraine headache with the use of vitamin C. Wishing to pass the information along to others, he described his experience in a letter which was published in the *London Daily Telegraph.*

"I only claim that I myself have found it beneficial," Mr. D. P. wrote. "I think that there are probably many cases of migraine and that there are probably other people who may find it [vitamin C] helpful. My doctor's reaction was that it could 'do no harm' and he was completely skeptical."

Mr. P. went on to say that he discovered the beneficial effects of vitamin C quite by accident:

"I had a severe migraine attack when it was necessary for me to do a lot of driving. In desperation I swallowed five 50 mgs. vitamin C tablets. Much to my surprise, the flashing lights and 'saw-edged' patterns disappeared within minutes and with no subsequent headache."

As a result of his letter, Mr. P. received a considerable amount of correspondence from his readers. He said, "This included two or three people who have thanked me, saying that their attacks have ceased within 30 minutes. I think it is also significant that grapefruit and grapefruit juice are effective. But orange juice has the opposite effect and makes the attacks worse. One of my correspondents has also found that lemon juice is helpful. Could it be that migraine is associated with a liver disorder?"

Note: If you decide to give vitamin C tablets a try, be sure to use those which are prepared from natural sources such as rose hips or acerola berries.

HERBAL REMEDIES FOR THE RELIEF OF MIGRAINE HEADACHE

Following are some of the ways in which migraine headache is treated with herbs. Proper diet of course is always advised along with the herbal medication.

Compound Herbal Formula

This prescription appeared in a work called *From a Practitioner's Case Book,* by H. Darwent, M.N.I.N.H.[3]

> In my opinion migraine is of organic origin; it is caused by the liver; this disturbs the sympathetic nervous system and its reaction brings on the severe headache in one particular region.
> I advise you to try this treatment:

> 1/2 oz. dandelion root
> 1/2 oz. centaury
> 1/2 oz. wild carrot *[Daucus carota]*
> 1/2 oz. ginger root
> 1/2 oz. marshmallow root
> 1/2 oz. motherwort
> 1/2 oz. vervain
> 1/4 oz. American mandrake root

> Mix all together and put half in two pints of water; bring to a boil and simmer for 15 minutes. Dose: Half a teacupful three times a day before meals. It should be a mild aperient [laxative] but senna [a laxative] can be added if required.
> This formula is a combination of liver and nerve herbs.
> The trouble will not go all at once; it will need steady perseverance for weeks. The period between attacks should lengthen and the severity reduce as the liver and nervous system gradually improve. Many sufferers have derived lasting benefit from this treatment.

Vervain Reported to Relieve Migraine

Vervain *(Verbena officinalis)* tea should not be overlooked in the search for freedom from the pain of migraine headache. Medical herbalists report that it has brought relief to many cases. One or two heaping teaspoonfuls of vervain is placed in a cup of boiling water. The tea is strained after it has cooled. One

---

[3] *Health from Herbs,* September-October 1967.

wineglassful (or more in severe cases) of the cold infusion is taken three or four times a day. We are told that it will not help in every case, but is perfectly harmless and well worth trying.

This interesting account on the use of vervain was submitted by a reader of *Grace* magazine:[4]

> I suffered from migraine for years, and it could not be cured. A copy of *Grace* was sent to my family in which vervain was mentioned for the relief of migraine. I insisted on trying it. After the first few cachets of dried vervain in my tea the migraine pains left me and have not been felt since.

Nature's Compress

A long-standing folk remedy for easing the pain of migraine is a cabbage leaf compress. One whole leaf or a few leaves with the large veins removed are crushed, then placed in a cloth and bound on the forehead at bedtime or when convenient during the day. The compress is renewed when the leaves dry out.

Various Methods of Coffee Therapy

Dr. J. E. Eichenlaub, M.D., suggests the use of coffee for relieving the pain of migraine headache: "Migraine or any other type of throbbing headache usually stems from engorged blood vessels. Strong coffee helps to shrink those vessels. One or two cups of strong coffee usually do enough good through this effect to make up for their jitters-spurring action. In severe attacks with nausea and vomiting, you sometimes can get relief by cooling a cup of strong coffee and taking it very slowly as an enema, retaining it as long as possible."[5]

Medical herbalists often recommend a very strong, hot coffee foot bath as a helpful measure for easing the pain of migraine.

Fringe Tree Famed as Migraine Remedy

The healing virtues of fringe tree *(Chionanthus virginicus)* were well known to the American Indians and early colonists. Frontier

---

[4]Summer 1968.

[5]*A Minnesota Doctor's Home Remedies for Common and Uncommon Ailments,* (Englewood Cliffs,N.J.:Prentice-Hall, Inc.,1960) p.123.

doctors boiled a tea from the bark and employed it as a headache remedy, especially for headaches of a bilious character.

In modern herbal medicine the rootbark of fringe tree is credited with having a specific influence on the liver. We are told that it liquifies the bile and helps to prevent the formation of gallstones. It is also considered among herbalists and homeopaths to be a valuable remedy for migraine headache.

A Case History

Mrs. Marjorie L. has written an account of her experiences with homeopathic Chionanthus (fringe tree). She says, "For over ten years I suffered frequent attacks of the most dreadful migraine headaches, accompanied by dizzy spells, nausea, vomiting of bile, and an overwhelming sense of depression. At first these bouts were occasional but as the years passed they came more often and lasted longer, until I only had about four or five days out of a month that I was not suffering from migraine. Although it is said that migraine is never fatal, I sometimes found myself wishing that it were. The many doctors I visited were unable to help me.

"Then one day I happened to read an article by a woman who claimed she had cured herself of migraine headaches with the use of homeopathic Chionanthus 6X. I confess that I really didn't think the remedy would help me, but I was desperate so I thought I'd give it a try. I sent for the preparation from a homeopathic pharmacy and took the tiny Chionanthus pellets according to the directions on the bottle.

"As the weeks passed I was amazed to find that the vicious migraine attacks were growing less violent and occurring far less often. And for the first time in years my dreadfully pale cheeks had some color and my eyes lost their dark sunken look. I could hardly believe the miracle that was happening!

"I have taken the Chionanthus remedy faithfully for several months now, and what a marvelous new lease on life it has given me! I can't praise it enough. I am entirely free of migraine headache and all its old horrors. No longer am I forced to spend all my days in bed. Instead I am now leading an active and happy existence once more. I often pause in my busy rounds these days to thank God for giving us the precious little fringe tree!"

NATURE'S REMEDIES
FOR COPING WITH OTHER FORMS OF HEADACHE

Because a healing method is old it does not follow that it is useless. Often the remedy of yesteryear becomes the top-line science of today. For example, a decoction of willow bark is an old-time remedy for muscular aches and for the pains of stiff joints, rheumatism, and headache. Today the synthetic drug most widely used as a specific for these conditions is aspirin. The chemical structure of aspirin is based on salicylic acid, a substance which scientists discovered in the willow bark!

Following are standard examples of the various methods employed by the family physicians of bygone days for treating various forms of headache. Many modern headache victims have found these remedies helpful. Perhaps you may too. The excerpts are from the book *Vitalogy,* by Drs. Wood and Ruddock:

Headache Remedies

1. To the juice of two large lemons add one quart of common table tea, made from the best green tea. Add the juice to the tea when the latter is boiling hot, and when cool bottle for use. Dose, one teacupful repeated in two or three hours.

2. Saturate a cloth with the tincture of witch hazel and apply to the part of the head where the pain is located; renew when the cloth becomes dry. Headache that is produced by an excessive flow of blood to the head, or is attended with the same, is usually cured with this remedy.

3. In many cases of headache, two teaspoonfuls of pulverized charcoal in half a teacupful of milk, will effectually relieve the patient in a very short period of time, more especially when there is acidity of the stomach. And in cases of costiveness many persons are cured by taking a tablespoonful three times a day. . . . Charcoal prepared from the young shoots of willow is preferable for most medical purposes.

(Note the reference to willow in this remedy).

Nervous Headaches

1. To a teacupful of water add one teaspoonful of the essence of peppermint; saturate a cloth with it and apply to the head and temples.

For many persons this will give very quick relief. As soon as the cloth becomes dry, wet the cloth again.

2. Wet a bunch of cotton or a piece of cotton cloth with camphor, roll it up and apply in the form of a compress to the back part of the head and the base of the brain. By means of a long strip of cloth carried over the top of the head, bind the compress tightly to its place; when it gets dry saturate it again with the camphor although one application will generally end the worst form of headache, especially when it occurs in the back part of the head.

3. When there are strong symptoms of an attack of nervous headache, drink freely, for three or four hours, of a strong decoction of scullcap. This will often effect a cure.

Sick Headache

This disease is frequently occasioned by deranged or unhealthy conditions of the stomach or liver.

Remedies:

1. When there are strong symptoms of sick headache, commence drinking lemon-water, prepared in the following manner: To two gills [half-pint] of tepid water, add one tablespoonful of the fresh juice of lemon, and drink this quantity every fifteen minutes, for one hour. Persons of strong constitution may add more of the lemon, or drink as much more water. This will produce a very salutary effect, and check or relieve it very materially.

2. Professor Sandborn of Montreal states that he has found hops to be an unfailing cure for sick headache, and found the same result with all others to whom he prescribed it. It is to be used as follows: Make a tea, and of that take a small teacupful every three hours; during a severe attack, every two hours. Drink it hot.

3. Guarana *(Paullinia sorbilis)* is an excellent remedy for sick headache. . . . Dose of the fluid extract, from ten drops to a teaspoonful. In headache, the dose may be repeated every half-hour or hour, until the pain ceases, though one dose is often sufficient. Professor Bundy, of the California Medical College, says, "When you have the headache, don't forget to take guarana." It is a favorite remedy with him, and he regards it as almost sure to relieve most forms of headache.

Note: Guarana is often called Brazilian cocoa because the flavor is remarkably similar to that of ordinary cocoa. According to South American legend, the stimulating action of this jungle vine was discovered by the Incas.

About 1/2 teaspoonful of guarana powder mixed in a little water makes a zesty beverage which the Brazilians drink for a "pick-up" in the afternoon during the hot seasons. They also use the beverage as a remedy for headaches resulting from depression or dissipation.

Now it is interesting to recall that Dr. Eichenlaub, a modern physician, recommends coffee for the relief of severe headache pain. Guarana contains more caffein than coffee (coffee about 0.5 to 2 percent; guarana 2.5 to 5 percent!) The caffein content apparently explains the effectiveness of guarana as a headache remedy.

Guarana of course should be avoided where coffee or tea are forbidden.

CHAPTER SUMMARY

1. Herbs are nature's remedies for coping with jittery nerves and nagging headache pain.
2. Botanicals used as nervines in domestic medicine are non-habit forming. They have a gentle soothing action and can be used over a long period of time, if necessary, without any ill effects.
3. There are a number of possible causes for the devastating attacks of migraine.
4. Many cases of migraine headache have been successfully treated with the use of plant medicine, or vitamin therapy.
5. Herbs are not outdated. That they contain the same healing virtues so well known to people of bygone days has been repeatedly demonstrated.

10

How Herbs Can Ease Your Foot Trouble

Foot miseries don't develop overnight. They are due in large part to self-torturing routines of shoe style and fashion—excessively high heels that double the weight on the forefoot—tight, binding shoes that force the feet out of shape causing them to bulge, throb, and burn—tight laces that cut deep into delicate tissues—non-porous shoe materials such as rubber or plastic that do not have the ability to "breathe," thereby producing the same effect as though the foot were locked in a steam chamber. So if your feet feel as though they are killing you, don't blame your barking "dogs" for deciding to bite back!

Cement pavement, hard floors, and certain occupations also contribute to foot discomfort. Policemen, letter carriers, nurses, dentists, salespeople, and others who walk or stand hours at a time on the job are frequently bothered with their feet.

And foot discomfort often makes you ache all over. When you limp to ease the pressure on your corn or bunion it puts an extra strain on your knee and hip, and in turn on various areas of your back. This may lead to headaches, backaches, and other unpleasant aches and pains. The practice of wearing high-heeled shoes can cause a similar reaction to take place as it alters the normal stance of the whole body.

Most of us cannot change our jobs just to ease our foot problems but we can provide preventive or corrective measures by purchasing better-fitting shoes and by devoting a little loving care to our feet at the end of a day's grind.

Your Shoes—Friend or Foe?

Five hundred women between the ages of 20 and 80 were examined by Dr. K. Sigg of Switzerland.[1] Of this number only ten had healthy feet, but among 200 male patients also examined, 40% had healthy feet. Many of the women complained of pains in the knee and hip joints as well as in the foot. Dr. Sigg blames these harmful effects on wearing the wrong kind of shoes, especially shoes with excessively high heels.

Corns, calluses, bunions, and plantar warts can be attributed to constricting shoes and high heels. Podiatrists (footcare specialists) have found that at whatever point a patient's toes were jammed into tight shoes, corns developed. And these specialists maintain that proper fitting shoes are a "must" before any treatment for corns can be expected to produce a lasting cure.

Early Foot Trouble

Foot trouble often begins during childhood when the feet are growing faster than the shoes wear out. In a foot health program of examining school children in Massachusetts, 75% of the youngsters were found to be wearing improperly fitted shoes. In England, a similar program revealed that 83% of the girls and 61% of the boys were wearing shoes that were too short.[2] Calluses and corns were almost universal in all the children over the age of ten.

Parents Take Heed

Parents are often unaware that their child may have foot problems. Often the child himself does not know. The bones of a youngster's feet are so pliable that he can squeeze his foot into shoes much too small with little difficulty. Even older children seldom complain that their feet hurt, even though wearing badly outgrown shoes and playing games in which the feet are put to hard use.

Here are some of the signs to watch for that may indicate the possibility that all is not well with your child's feet: He removes

---

[1] *Consumer Bulletin,* August 1968.

[2] *Medical Press.*

his shoes and socks at every chance he gets; he seems unusually clumsy, and trips and falls more frequently than most children of his age; he tends to stop playing and sits down; he tells you his legs hurt. If he does any of these things it would be a good idea to inspect his feet carefully for blisters, corns, etc., and to check his shoes and socks to see whether or not he has outgrown them. (Ill-fitting shoes or stockings can ruin growing feet.) And it would be very wise to have his feet examined by a podiatrist.

Actually a parent should not wait until such indications become obvious. It would be far better to keep an ever-watchful eye on your child's feet, and take him to a foot specialist for a check-up at regular intervals.

SOME BASIC FOOT-CARE RULES FOR ALL

Here are some of the basic rules podiatrists suggest to help keep your feet in good condition:

1. Wash the feet every day, but do not use strong detergent soaps. Use a mild soap such as castile for example, and warm, not hot water.
2. Dry the feet by patting gently with a towel.
3. Do not cut ingrown toenails, corns, or calluses.
4. For dry skin apply cocoa butter or olive oil.
5. Exercise your feet—do some walking.
6. Toe straight ahead when walking. Pointing the toes out or in throws the body out of line.
7. Give your feet a breath of fresh air. Walk barefoot on a clean beach or on a carpet of clean unsprayed lawn.
8. Be sure your hose and shoes fit properly.
9. Genuine leather is considered the ideal shoe material. Because of its porous nature, leather allows the feet to breathe and this helps foot sweat to evaporate rapidly. It is resilient, yet strong enough to give the necessary support. Tests have proved that leather soles are four times as resistant to punctures as any other type of shoe material. This gives you far greater protection should you accidently step on a nail, tack, or other sharp object. Leather soles absorb the shock waves from continuous

pounding on pavement, hard floors, and concrete steps, rather than passing the shocks on to your tender feet.

10. Purchase your shoes after you've been on your feet all day, as your feet will be more sensitive at this time.

11. New shoes should be broken in carefully and slowly. At first, wear them only a few hours each day.

12. Inspect the feet regularly, checking for corns, calluses, blisters, etc.

13. If an ulcer or sore occurs on the leg or foot seek professional help.

14. Clean the toenails carefully, using an orange stick; do not use metal.

15. Check the linings of your shoes frequently for ravels, rough spots, or tears.

16. Do not wear tight garters or socks that have tight elastic bands.

17. Always trim the toenails by cutting straight across, not curved. After trimming, smooth with an emery board.

18. Replace your child's shoes with a larger size the moment it is indicated. When purchasing his socks, allow for 1/4 inch beyond the end of the longest toe.

19. Exercise the feet as it helps restore strength and tone to the muscles. Here are some suggestions: Sit in a straight-backed chair and remove your shoes and stockings. Extend your legs and flex the toes rapidly up and down for about 30 seconds to one minute. Now move the feet forward and backward as far as they will go, then rotate the feet and move them from side to side. Practice picking up a marble or pencil with the toes (about ten times) to give the toes strength and agility.

HERBAL AIDS TO HELP YOU WALK IN PEACE

Herbal aids can also do much to help you achieve the goal of happy feet. The following natural remedies have been used by many people in all parts of the world to obtain blessed relief from foot discomfort that would otherwise take the joy out of a beautiful day.

How to Relieve Pain of Corns and Calluses

1. Soak the feet in warm water just before bedtime. After they are carefully dried, apply lemon juice to the corn. Repeat the treatment nightly until results are obtained.
2. Another method advises keeping the corn well saturated with castor oil until it softens and disappears.
3. Fresh, not canned, pineapple has a solid reputation as a natural corn remover. Bind a small piece of the peel (the inner side) to the corn with a band-aid. Leave it on overnight. Remove in the morning and soak the foot in fairly hot water. The corn can then be easily removed.
4. For soft corns between the toes, cover with a soft cloth saturated with oil of wintergreen night and morning for several days.
5 A foot bath of yarrow leaves has been found helpful for the relief of calluses and corns. To prepare, add one cup of yarrow leaves and one tablespoonful of salt to three quarts of boiling water. Turn off the burner immediately, then cover the container and allow the infusion to stand until the heat is reduced to a comfortable degree. Strain off the herb and soak your feet in the herbal water. Repeat each day as needed.
6. Calluses may be softened by frequent applications of either olive oil, sesame seed oil, castor oil, or wheat germ oil.

Plantar Warts

A wart that develops on the bottom of the foot is called a plantar wart. This type is more deeply imbedded than warts that appear on other areas of the body.

External applications of wheat germ oil or castor oil are reputed to disperse plantar warts. A pad of cotton saturated with the oil is bound on the wart at bedtime and allowed to remain on overnight. This is repeated nightly until results are achieved (generally about three or four weeks).

Cracks on the Heels

Apply sunflower seed oil frequently to the heels. To prevent a recurrence of the trouble, apply the oil occasionally.

Coping with Athlete's Foot Infection

The burning, itching condition of athlete's foot, probably the most common of all fungus infections, is caused by the presence of a tiny microorganism. It may occur at any time; however, it is more prevalent in hot weather.

There are several things which can contribute to getting the infection: profuse sweating of the feet; uncleanliness; friction of the stockings and shoes against the feet; direct contact with the fungus (for example, stepping into a shower that has been used by someone who has athlete's foot).

Because of its contagious nature, this fungus infection can spread to other areas of the body, such as the hands and face, due to contact with the original site.

Suggested Remedy: Use a soft brush and wash the feet thoroughly but lightly with mild soap and warm water. Work up a good lather and continue washing the feet for about five or ten minutes, then rinse and pat dry. Now apply apple cider vinegar to the feet, making sure to get the areas in between the toes. This precedure should be followed nightly until the condition clears.

Further Instructions: Change the stockings often, at least once a day, and use a fresh towel for drying the feet after each foot bath. To prevent reinfection through the soiled socks and towels, boil them for 15 minutes. The socks may then be soaked in a solution of one-fourth cup of white vinegar to one gallon of cold water. Do not rinse, but simply squeeze and hang them in the sun to dry. The vinegar solution is excellent for removing the unpleasant odor of soiled stockings and will give them a fresh clean smell.

Alternate Remedy for Athlete's Foot

Many people claim good results from using red clover blossoms as a remedy for athlete's foot. One cup of the blossoms is boiled until thick. When the pulp has cooled it is bound on the affected parts after the feet have been thoroughly washed. This is done every night until the unpleasant condition is eliminated.

Herbal Foot Baths

Plunging your tired, burning feet into an old-fashioned herbal foot bath at the end of a weary day is one of the most soothing things you can do. The botanicals for these baths may be used singularly or two or three may be used in combination. Rosemary, eucalyptus leaves, oat straw, mugwort, low-mallow, camomile, and meadowsweet are among the many herbs that may be employed.

Directions:
1. Place about two or three handfuls of the herb or combination of herbs in one gallon of boiling water; cover and allow the mixture to cool to the warmth most comfortable for a foot bath. Strain off the herb and soak the feet for 15 or 20 minutes, reheating the herbal water as required.
2. An excellent foot bath can be made by simply adding a teaspoonful of pine oil to one gallon of warm water.

The Alternate Foot Bath

The alternate method—soaking the feet in very warm herbal water, then in cold herbal water—is a refreshing tonic which stimulates the circulation and makes your toes tingle with joy. It also soothes swollen ankles after you've been on your feet all day.

Directions: Prepare enough of the herbal infusion (according to previous directions) to make two separate foot baths. Pour half of the infusion into a container and allow it to become cold. The other half should be kept quite warm. Soak the feet for five minutes in the warm foot bath, then immediately plunge them into the cold foot bath for one minute, then back into the warm. Alternate four or five times, ending with the cold foot bath. Then dry the feet thoroughly.

Soothing Herbal Foot Powders

Here is a wonderful dusting powder you can use for hot, tired, aching feet. This is an especially welcome herbal aid during the warm weather. Mix together equal parts of powdered slippery elm, bayberry bark, and golden seal. Dust the feet as needed or sprinkle the powder in the socks. You will be delighted with the soothing results.

Eliminating Strong Foot Odor

Wash the feet in mild soap and warm water. Rinse. Apply apple cider vinegar straight or diluted.

Socks should be changed often. To deodorize the soiled stockings, soak them in a solution of white vinegar and water directly after they have been given a thorough washing.

Excessive Sweating of the Feet

Sweating of the feet is normal but excessive sweating can cause trouble.

Tips to help keep your feet dry: The feet should be bathed often and the stockings changed at least once a day. Cotton socks or socks with cotton soles are absorbent and can be worn with good results. Wearing leather shoes is also helpful as leather allows the air to circulate around the feet. Witch hazel applied to the bottoms of the feet will reduce excessive foot perspiration. Herbal foot dusting powders used after bathing is another valuable aid.

Cold Feet

This condition is generally caused by dampness or poor circulation.

Cork insoles or shoes made of similar absorbent material should not be worn as they retain moisture. Leather affords protection against dampness and helps keep the feet dry and comfortable. Another plan is to wear two pairs of stockings of different material—wool, and cotton or silk. The cotton or silk should be worn next to the skin and the woolen pair over them.

Since the alternate foot bath stimulates circulation, it can be used with good effect for relieving the condition of cold feet.

Circulation can also be improved by good nutrition, especially including the use of vitamin E. The value of this vitamin for circulatory troubles has been repeatedly demonstrated. You will get vitamin E if you include lots of natural wheat germ and plenty of vegetable oils and salads in your diet. Otherwise your diet can be supplemented with vitamin E capsules.

Varicose Veins—Phlebitis

A medical journal[3] reported that 44 patients suffering from various types of varicose veins were treated daily with 300 to 500 milligrams of vitamin E for from two months to three years. Seven of the cases were completely healed; nine showed improvement within one month; the rest showed improvement and experienced some relief from pain, edema, and congestion. No side effects were observed.

In the magazine *Attivita Congresso degli Cariologia,*[4] the writers mentioned five cases of acute phlebitis which healed quickly with vitamin E therapy. Another report[5] discussed four cases of phlebitis treated only with vitamin E in which inflammation subsided and the swelling disappeared.

Bunions

Shoes that are too narrow at the forefoot cause pressure at the big toe joint. This irritates the bursal sac and causes swelling that gradually results in the painful disability known as a bunion. When high heels are worn, more weight is placed on the front part of the foot and makes the bunion worse.

If the condition is in the very early stage where the irritation has only just become noticeable, a foot bath prepared with comfrey root will help relieve the inflammation. Place two handfuls of the cut root in one gallon of water and boil slowly for 30 minutes. Then strain and allow the decoction to cool to a comfortable warmth. Soak the foot in the comfrey water for 10 or 15 minutes morning and night.

Stick to shoes with low or medium heels, and be certain the shoes are wide enough at the forefoot.

---

[3]*La Riforma Medical,* (1955).

[4]May 1948.

[5]*Surgery,* Vol. 28, 1950.

Ingrown Toenail

This condition generally results from improper toenail cutting, or from narrow pointed shoes, or from shoes or stockings that are too tight. To prevent the condition, podiatrists recommend proper footwear, and also advise that the nails always be trimmed by cutting straight across, not curved down into the corners and not shorter than the length of the toes. After trimming, the nails should be smoothed with an emery board.

For temporary relief of the inflammation caused by ingrown toenail, medical herbalists suggest that the foot be soaked in a warm comfrey root foot bath for 20 minutes, two or three times a day.

Be sure to have the ingrown toenail trimmed by a podiatrist as soon as possible.

Chilblains

This is a condition in which the skin becomes inflammed and itches intensely. Frequent applications of lemon juice mixed with glycerine have proved successful in clearing up chilblains.

Comfrey Root Tea for Gout

This painful condition, characterized by swelling or inflammation about a joint, is due to excess uric acid in the blood. The big toe joint is a frequent site for the deposits of urates.

Medical herbalists have reported good results in treating gout with comfrey root tea. One-half to one ounce of the cut root is boiled in one quart of water for half an hour. It is then strained and a wineglassful of the decoction is taken three times a day.

Fallen Arches

Village healers in some parts of the world treat the condition of fallen arches with a liniment made from the herb wormwood. This is prepared by adding one ounce of powdered wormwood to a pint of rum and allowing the mixture to stand for one week, shaking the bottle thoroughly every night. At the end of the week the liquid is strained off and placed in a tightly capped bottle. The liniment is rubbed on the feet night and morning, and in between times the foot is kept bound with gauze. It is said that beneficial results are generally obtained in about three or four weeks.

Cramps in the Foot or Leg

Although the excruciatingly painful cramp in the leg or foot that awakens many a person during the night may arise from a serious disturbance, doctors find that the usual simple cause is a deficiency of calcium. And in some cases where an individual does get enough of this mineral, his body may not be assimilating it properly due to a lack of vitamin D. Nutritionalists explain that vitamin D is necessary for the utilization of calcium.

Nocturnal leg and foot cramps might also be caused by a mild deficiency or faulty utilization of vitamin E. This possibility was discovered by accident when Drs. Mahan and Ayers of Los Angeles successfully treated a number of patients with vitamin E for obstinate skin conditions. Both doctors said that several patients had mentioned suffering from severe nocturnal leg cramping but that after taking the vitamin E for their skin trouble their painful leg cramps ceased![6] Encouraged by these results, the medics treated 26 patients troubled with leg cramps by giving them 100 I.U. of d-alpha-tocopherol acetate three times a day before meals. Of the 26 patients, 22 obtained excellent results and four reported moderate improvement. Relief from painful cramping was prompt, generally within one or two weeks. Two of the patients stopped taking the vitamin E after about eight weeks, and within a month or five weeks later both were suffering again from leg cramps.

The British medical journal *Lancet* also reports that vitamin E has been found helpful in relieving cramps of the legs.

Other Treatments: Here are some of the treatments others have employed for relieving the condition of leg or foot cramps:

1. An issue of the *Organic Consumer Report*[7] states that troublesome muscular cramps occurring most often at night "can

---

[6]*California Medicine,* August 1969.

[7]September 1, 1964.

be relieved in 15 or 20 minutes through the use of a tablespoon of calcium lactate[8] taken with one teaspoon each of cider vinegar and honey in hot water."

2. The famed Dr. Jarvis has found that honey helps to relieve the condition of muscle cramps. He suggests two teaspoons of honey at each meal. Or the honey may be combined with two teaspoonfuls of apple cider vinegar in a glass of water.

3. The bark of the high cranberry bush *(Viburnum opulus)* is an old-time favorite for relieving cramps. This plant was well known to the American Indians. In his book, *Indian Household Medicine Guide,* John Lighthall wrote that high cranberry "is usually called cramp-bark from the fact that it is such a powerful antispasmodic, and is noted for subduing cramps so readily." He recommended the hot tea for severe cramps, "a big swallow every three or four hours." For milder cases, "a dose of the tincture, from 10 to 30 drops three or four times a day."

High cranberry bark was also a favorite of the horse and buggy doctors. Physicians Wood and Ruddock wrote: "Make a strong tea of the high cranberry bush bark, and drink one-third of a teacupful and it will stop the cramp in 20 minutes." To prevent a recurrence of the trouble they suggested drinking the tea night and morning for one or two weeks.

4. Many people use red raspberry leaf tea as a domestic remedy for preventing cramps in the legs if caused by poor circulation. The tea is taken night and morning. It is said that if the tea is discontinued, the cramps will generally return again within a few days.

CHAPTER SUMMARY

1. Use herbs for treatment of corns and calluses.
2. Specific herbs and herbal products provide natural and effective ways of coping with a large variety of foot pain problems.
3. Refreshing and soothing foot baths can be made with herbs, either singly or in combination.
4. Herbal foot powders are a welcome aid, especially during the hot weather.
5. Herbal remedies can relieve the torturous pain of nocturnal foot and leg cramps.

---

[8]A food supplement obtainable from drug and health food stores.

11

How Herbs Can Help Shed
Unwanted Pounds

If you are overweight, do you find yourself on a perpetual merry-go-round of low-calorie austerity and high-calorie eating binges? Instead of hating yourself for not getting off this merry-go-round, why not try herbal aids? They could make things much easier for you in losing excess weight.

The use of herbs is primarily a matter of personalized slimming—finding the right formula that works best for you, personally. However, on an overall basis all herbal aids which have stood the test of time generally produce good results for almost everyone.

CLEAVERS: HERBAL SLIMMING SECRET OF THE ANCIENTS

There are numerous herbs and plant products which have a longstanding reputation for trimming the figure. Cleavers *(Galium aparine)*, which the Chinese call *Chu-yang-yang*, is a classic example. It was considered by the ancients an excellent remedy for obesity and also for cleansing the blood.

In modern botanic medicine, cleavers is classed as an alterative (changing nutritive processes of the body), diuretic (kidney stimulant), aperient (bowel stimulant), and tonic.

How a Woman Shed 32 Pounds

A medical herbalist reported the case of an overweight woman who took daily infusions of cleavers. During the first month nothing happened, but then on the fifth week she began slowly losing weight, and at the end of six months her weight was down to normal. She had lost a total of 32 pounds and has not put them back on again.

How to Prepare Cleavers for Reducing

To make an infusion of cleavers, you simply put a teaspoonful of the herb in a teacup and pour on boiling water. Cover and let stand for 15 minutes, then strain and drink hot or cold—one teacupful three times a day between meals.

THE WEIGHT-REDUCING POWER OF FENNEL

Fennel, popular as a culinary herb, has the added distinction of being regarded as a slimming aid and strengthener of the eyes. In 1657, William Coles wrote, "Both the seeds, leaves, and roots of our garden fennel are much used in drinks and broths for those that are grown fat, to abate their unwieldiness and cause them to grow more gaunt and lank." John Evelyn mentioned that country women made the herb into broths and teas for slimming.

It is believed that the ancient Greeks were well acquainted with the weight-reducing power of this herb, as the Greek name for fennel is *Marathron,* which is derived from *Mariano,* "to grow thin."

How One Woman Reduced with Fennel Seed Tea

One lady reported that she brought her weight down from 210 to 140 lbs. after several months of consistent use of fennel seed tea. She said, "I always drank four cups of the tea each day, one before breakfast, one on my 'coffee break,' one before dinner, and one just before going to bed. I did not follow a strict diet but just cut down a little on the starches, sugars, and fats. Besides losing weight, I received an unexpected health benefit. I had never heard that fennel was good for the eyes, but after only two and a half months of drinking the tea I noticed that an old eye discomfort (bright light pained my eyes) had disappeared." (*Note:* Fennel is a member of the parsley herb family and is rich in vitamin A.)

How to Prepare Fennel Seed Tea

To prepare fennel seed tea, put four teaspoonfuls of the seeds in two pints of boiling water and simmer for five minutes. Remove from the burner, keep the container covered, and allow to stand for 15 minutes, then strain. The tea is now ready for use—one teacupful three or four times daily. It may be reheated if desired.

Dieter Praises Fennel Seed in Powdered Form

Another woman claimed excellent results with the use of fennel seed in *powdered* form. She tells us she put the powder in capsules and took two capsules four times a day. "I had a very stubborn weight problem," she said, "and tried dieting many times. I'd lose a few pounds at first, then for two or three weeks at a stretch I'd not lose another ounce even though I still followed my diet religiously. It was always at this point that my poor will power would just give out and I'd start eating everything again.

"Then one day a friend suggested I try powdered fennel seed. I don't know if it would help others with a stubborn weight problem but it certainly did marvels for me. When I went back on my diet and took the capsules of powdered fennel seed my weight dropped steadily—no more episodes of trying to struggle through periods where the pounds just wouldn't come off. I have been down to my normal weight for some time now and I find that I can be fairly liberal in my eating habits without gaining, so long as I keep taking my capsules of powdered fennel seed. I have also noticed that fennel has done wonders for my digestion."

Some of the herb companies carry powdered fennel seed in capsule form.

KELP: REDUCING AID FROM THE SEA

Obesity (overweight) is seldom seen among the Polynesians and other races who use seaweeds as a regular part of their daily diet.

One of the most commonly known seaweeds is kelp (*Fucus vesiculosis*), also called bladderwrack.

Kelp's Reputation As an Anti-Fat Worker

T. J. Lyle, M.D., writes:[1]

This plant [kelp] has a reputation as an anti-fat, claiming that it diminishes fat without in any respect injuring the health. It influences the mucous membranes and the lymphatics. It is a gently stimulating and toning alterant. It is one of those slow, persistent agents that require time to accomplish the desired results. It is stimulating to the absorbents and especially influences the fatty globules. Its best action is observed in individuals having a cold, torpid, clammy skin and loose flabby rolls of fat.

Dr. Eric Powell has this to say about kelp: "Fucus, or kelp as it is known, is an old remedy for obesity, and is probably still the best. Its action on fatty tissue is mainly due to its iodine content and the association of that element with the thyroid gland. But we also know that Fucus acts directly on the fat cells. It has a regulating effect, and while it aids in the reduction of fat, it may be taken with perfect safety by the thin, as it is a *normalizer.*"

Infusions of kelp are particularly slimy and unpleasant tasting, so few people can face drinking them. Fortunately, however, kelp can be obtained in tablet form from herb companies or health food stores.

HOW LECITHIN ATTACKS THOSE STUBBORN FAT BULGES

Lecithin, derived mainly from soybeans, should be included in every weight-watcher's program. Lecithin helps control the figure as it pulls the fat deposits from stubborn fat bulges in your body and "burns" them out. These are the fat areas you so often wished would melt away. Lecithin also helps you feel well-fed on less food so you're not tempted to indulge in overeating or nibbling between meals.

There is evidence that lecithin also helps prevent many health problems like cholesterol build-up and gall bladder complications, and further that it increases energy and brain power.

Lecithin in various forms—capsules, granules, or liquid—are all available from your health food store or herb company.

---

[1]*Physio-Medical Therapeutics, Materia Medica and Pharmacy.*

RASPBERRY LEAVES: ANOTHER POPULAR REDUCING AID

In his article which appeared in a health publication, Martin Thoresby says, "One of the most successful herbs for acquisition of a good figure, and in controlling it, is raspberry leaves." He mentions that some time ago it was revealed that in Japan, girls on a training program for figure improvement were given daily infusions of raspberry leaf tea as part of their training course, "and results were said to be 'miraculous' at the end of one month."

A Super Figure

Thoresby also includes this interesting bit of information: "The writer once worked alongside a girl who had a super figure—at least the men thought so! Her secret was to take raspberry leaf infusion three times daily between meals, and she adhered to this therapy even at the office. As a result, in combination with a mile walk daily (walking slowly, head erect, tummy in, chest out), she entered a local beauty contest and won even at the age of 39, and in competition with over 100 entrants many of whom were 'safe bets' that they would gain the title."

Raspberry Leaves Combined with Kelp Results in Model Figure

"Another girl," continues Thoresby, "over a period of two months, slimmed to the extent that she was known as 'the slimmest girl in the organization,' and there were some pretty slim girls too. Apart from a daily intake of honey her secret was to drink raspberry leaf infusion twice daily and take two tablets of Bladderwrack morning and night. She reached the stage where she even became a model for a fashion house."

SLIMMING THE HONEY WAY

Honey taken by itself (not mixed with other foods) is an age-old remedy for obesity, and is still popular today. Thoresby says: "It is possible to slim the honey way. Having recommended it to many women I have found that considerable weight reduction is possible at a dosage of two dessertspoonfuls daily."

SLIMMING THE GRAPE JUICE WAY

Another popular aid for reducing is grape juice. This natural health drink is also one of nature's finest blood cleansers.

Slimming Secrets of a Famous Mystic

The late Edgar Cayce, famed "Sleeping Prophet" of Virginia Beach, mentioned the use of grape juice as a reducing aid. Here are a few extracts from his readings while in a psychic trance:[2]

Obesity: Female, 18 years old. No.1431-2 3/24/51

Q.-5 How can I reduce safely, and how much should I weigh?
A.-5 About a hundred and fifty pounds. Reduce by the grape juice way.
Q.-6 Please outline the diet.
A.-6 Eat anything you like, save potatoes and white bread. But take four glasses of grape juice each day—half an hour before the meals and before retiring. This would be three-quarters of a glass of the grape juice and one-quarter of plain water stirred together. Take about five to ten minutes to drink the juice each time, see?

Obesity: Tendencies. Male, 47 years old. No. 1589-1 5/13/38

Before the morning and the evening meals, about half an hour before, take at least two ounces of grape juice—in one ounce of plain water; not charged water. This will prevent the body taking on weight, and will make for nearer normal weight for the body.

If there are not too much sugars, nor too much of any drinks that are fermented, these will be the necessary combinations for the correcting of the condition.

Appetite: Obesity. Female, 56 years old. No. 1309-2 4/10/40

Take grape juice four times each day; one ounce of plain water and three ounces of grape juice, taken half an hour before each meal and upon retiring. Then in the matter of the diet, it will almost take care of itself, and take those things the appetite calls for, save sweets, chocolate or the like; not great quantities of sugars, nor of pastries; but all other

---

[2]From the files of the Association for Research and Enlightenment, Incorporated, Virginia Beach, Va. 23451.

foods, vegetables or meats, provided they are not fats, may be taken according to the appetite; but we will find the appetite will change a a great deal.

Obesity: Tendencies. Male, 51 years old. No. 470-32 4/4/41

As to the increase in weight—this may be controlled by the grape juice way, rather than any particular dieting; just requiring that the body refrain from too much sweets and starches.

SWITCH FROM SALT TO THE MAGIC OF HERBS

Restricting salt is an easy way to trim your figure and accrue big dividends in health benefits at the same time.

Salt attracts and holds water in the body; just one teaspoonful of salt, for example, will retain three quarts of water in the tissues of your body. So if you want to lose weight with very little effort, simply toss away your salt shaker and you may shed as much as three pounds the first week. Of course you must also avoid foods that have been salted such as potato chips, pretzels, salted peanuts, salted crackers, salted cheeses, and foods that are preserved in salt like ham, bacon, pickles, relishes, certain types of sausages, etc. Artificially softened water should also be shunned because of its high sodium content. Your body can get all the vital food salts it needs for your well-being from fruits, vegetables, and meats in their natural state.

Remember, too, that salt makes you thirsty so you are bound to drink more water which means more weight. A person can carry one to one and a half gallons of water due to the salt that is in the body.

When you kick the salt habit you will shed liquid weight, not fat. However, eliminating salt will greatly help you in your battle to reduce the bulges of fat too, for salt is a stimulant and excites the appetite by increasing the flow of saliva, thus creating a greater desire for food.

Salt—a Health Hazard

Excessive salt intake not only is an enemy to slimming, but also has an adverse effect on the health. Sinus trouble, heart and kidney disease, high blood pressure, strokes, asthma, headaches, and insomnia are some of the many conditions that seem to result from eating too much salt.

For example, Dr. John H. Laragh, professor of clinical medicine at Columbia University College of Physicians and Surgeons, said that a striking fact about high blood pressure "is its close relationship to the amount of salt that a patient eats. There's no question, both in experimental animals and in humans, that increased dietary salt consumption in various parts of the world is associated with much more high blood pressure and with a higher incidence of strokes. Conversely, there's no question about the beneficial effect of withholding salt from the diet of patients with high blood pressure."

Dr. Laragh suggests that the reason salt raises the blood pressure is that it "creates a hydraulic effect by retaining fluid in the circuit, and this in turn tends *per se* to raise blood pressure." In short, a large volume of fluid requires more pressure to circulate, besides adding excess body weight.

Herbs—Your Zesty Flavor Substitutes for Salt

No need to worry about meals tasting flat without salt. Just switch to zesty, flavorful herbs as recommended below and you'll enjoy some delightful adventures in new taste sensations. It's fun to experiment with do-it-yourself seasoning with herbs and spices—ginger, rosemary, oregano, tarragon, cloves, sage, allspice, caraway, dill, and a host of others. A good rule to follow is to use just a little of these natural seasoners at first, particularly if a new flavor. You can always add more to suit your taste but it is almost impossible to remove or correct seasoning if too much has been initially used. And use of these herbs adds nothing to body weight by retaining water in the tissues.

How to Use Nature's Flavor Magic

Here are a few suggestions for adding nature's flavor magic to your diet. In place of salt, sprinkle a little oregano, paprika, or tarragon on your eggs. If you put salt on your tomatoes, try a dash of basil instead. You can season roasts with pepper, ground rosemary, or ginger before cooking; flavor veal with powdered mint or cayenne; for green beans try savory or chili powder; use either dill, marjoram, or bay leaves for stews; ground allspice may be sprinkled on sweet potatoes or squash.

Curry powder, a subtle mixture of exotic herbs and spices of the Far East, can be used for meats, fish, eggs, vegetables, mushrooms, soups and sauces. And you might try saffron, a true gourmet flavoring for seafood salads, scrambled eggs, soups, and fish sauces. Caraway seeds add greatly to the flavor of soup stock, stewed meats, and sauerkraut. Basil, called "Herb of the King" by ancient Greeks, is widely known today as the tomato herb and may be used for flavoring meat loaf and all tomato recipes.

When you set your dinner table, include little containers of different herbs and spices which offer never-ending pleasures of taste, and invite your family to go creative. They'll attain unknown heights of flavor variety.

The switch from salt to the magic of herbs will increase your go-power, and you'll be thrilled to see your figure gradually slimming down normally, and in the right places!

CHAPTER SUMMARY

1. Herbs are inexpensive, personalized reducing aids, but remember they work slowly and constructively.
2. Herbal aids are not dangerous drugs; there is no strain on the system or drain on the health in reducing body weight.
3. Along with their slimming power, certain herbs and plant products contribute various health benefits (e.g., cleanse the blood, strengthen the eyes, assist digestion, reduce or prevent cholesterol deposits), thereby increasing your go-power while decreasing your girth.
4. Lecithin helps to normalize the body that is heavy in spots. It also lessens hunger pangs and in this way helps remove the temptation to overeat or to snack between meals.
5. Evidence indicates that excessive intake of salt is a health hazard as well as an enemy to slimming.
6. Restricting salt in the diet, substituting tasty herbs, is an easy way to lose weight.

12

How to Use Herbs for Youthful Skin and Complexion

Women have always continued to seek ways to remove those facial wrinkles and to give their complexion that irresistible "come-hither look." Back in the eras of ancient splendor, famous beauties attributed the longevity of their youthful skin tone to the use of herbal formulas. Then came the synthetic age with high pressure advertising, and the wonderland of nature was all but forgotten. Women became imbued with the idea that chemical laboratories could solve all cosmetic problems, and in record-breaking time at that.

Now the pendulum is swinging the other way again. In many parts of the world, do-it-yourself methods utilizing herbs and natural foods for skin health and beauty are becoming tremendously popular. There are many reasons for this. Every modern woman, like her ancient counterpart, wants lovely skin, but in her search for beauty she has learned that many commercial creams that promise a glowing complexion contain hormones, antibiotics, or other irritants that do more harm than good.

Adverse effects can be so slight that they may go unnoticed, or take several days or longer to develop. Cosmetic reactions may appear as dryness, skin cracking, swelling, itchiness or rashes. Fortunately, a few experts within the beauty business are becoming concerned about the side-effects which can result from synthetic formulations and are starting to look to nature for better ingredients.

Another reason for the growing interest in home-preparations of natural beauty aids is the money-saving angle. Compared to the more than 2½ billion dollars American women have been spending each year for commercial beauty products, herbs cost next to nothing. And women are also finding out that an added incentive for being their own beauticians is that natural ingredients are often more effective.

What Cosmetic Herbs Can Do for You

In terms of beauty, herbs can help tone up the tissues, smooth away wrinkles and impart a quality of softness to dry leathery skin. Oversized pores that give the complexion a pitted look can be reduced with the help of botanicals. There are herbs that can stimulate the areas of poor circulation and bring a flush of healthy activity to the complexion. Others dig deep to lift large amounts of grime from the pores, and help banish that aging skin appearance. Still others can improve skin troubled by oil gland problems. These are only a few of the many ways herbs can help bring out the hidden beauty of your skin.

WHAT YOU SHOULD KNOW ABOUT YOUR SKIN

Your skin is a vital complex organ, not just a strong envelope to keep you in and everything else out. As an organ of sensation or touch it is closely connected to the great nerve centers of your body. It is composed of more or less 20 square feet of specialized tissue for the average-sized person, and has many life-preserving functions. As a temperature regulator it helps prevent the loss of heat when you are exposed to a cold environment. In over-heated bodily conditions resulting from hot surroundings, fevers, or strenuous exercises, the skin relieves your tissues by helping the heat to escape through profuse sweating. Sweating is also a response to sudden emotional stress or fear.

How Your Skin Stays Healthy

Your skin maintains its health by excreting sebum, a fatty substance which oozes to the surface where it forms a special kind of mixture with sweat. This helps keep your skin pliable and moist. In very cold weather the sebum often congeals as it reaches the surface; when this occurs your skin dries and chaps. And this also happens occasionally when your hands are not thoroughly dried after being in water.

Skin Changes

Overproduction or underproduction of the sebum can cause excessively dry or oily skin. At puberty the sex hormones affect the skin through the blood stream and stimulate the sebaceous glands. This sudden increase of sebum activity may clog the pores and cause blackheads, pimples, or other skin distresses. In premature aging the sebum production slacks off considerably, causing the skin fibres to lose much of their tone and elasticity. The result is dry, wrinkled, leathery skin.

Your Protective Acid Mantle

The surface of your skin is normally acid, and this protective covering has been given the name *acid mantle*. It acts as a barrier against bacterial invasion. When you wash yourself with harsh alkaline soaps you also wash off your protective acid mantle and it takes many hours before your body can restore it.

Skin As A Built-In Purifier

Your skin "breathes," drawing in oxygen and exhaling impurities. A great portion of the waste is discharged in the form of invisible gases called *insensible perspiration*. And whether or not you are aware of it, this process continues steadily day and night. A lesser amount of toxins is excreted in the form of visible perspiration, which generally collects like tiny beads or droplets on the surface of your skin.

Often the skin will assume an increased burden of elimination in order to relieve the work-load of some distressed organ, as in the case of weak kidneys or decreased liver function, and to a lesser degree when the lungs are not working adequately. Toxins from the bowels are sometimes eliminated through the skin.

Were it not for these remarkable arrangements of removing vicious poisons from the body, the blood would become so polluted it would no longer be able to support life.

The Process of Absorption

Another function nature has allotted to your skin is the ability to absorb certain external substances such as ointments or lotions that are applied to it. However, this absorption factor also means that unless your skin is properly bathed and cared for, the impurities deposited on its surface through perspiration accumulate and the waste may be reabsorbed into your body, causing the system to become toxic.

Layers of the Skin

Your skin is composed of four layers which are constantly being renewed. The surface layer (epidermis) flakes off and depends upon the layers underneath for its constant renewal. That is why it is important (1) to use a little friction when bathing, so that the dead-flaking cells can be thoroughly removed, allowing the tissues underneath to breath; and (2) to use cosmetics sparingly, also taking care never to apply fresh make-up over the stale. If these two rules, along with that of cleanliness, are not followed there is trouble in the form of clogged pores and rough, crepy skin that cannot breathe.

DO-IT-YOURSELF HERBAL BEAUTY AIDS

The all-time favorite herbal ingredients of the beauty recipes that follow are available to everyone—easy to use, easy to prepare, and costing but a few cents. It doesn't matter which you select so long as it meets your own personal beauty needs.

When preparing your herbal ingredients *do not* use an aluminum container. Use either Pyrex or enamelware. *This is very important.*

One more point should be noted. Some recipes call for the use of a cloth dipped into the herbal solution, then applied to the face. Be sure the cloths are fresh, and keep them aside to be used only for your facial beauty treatments.

HERBAL SKIN CLEANSERS AND CONDITIONERS

Tropical Cleansing Delight

This treatment is to be used only once a week.

Place a papaya tea bag in one pint of boiling water. Cover and allow the tea to simmer for a few minutes, then remove from the burner and let it stand until the heat is noticeably reduced. Toss out the tea bag and pour the solution into a porcelain or Pyrex bowl. Place two white washcloths into the liquid; wring out one of the cloths loosely and apply it to your face. To retain the heat as long as possible you can either fold the cloth or place a dry towel over it.

When the cloth begins to lose its heat, replace it in the tea and immediately wring out the second cloth and hold it on your face. The papaya solution must be kept reasonably hot so that the pores of the skin can remain open and the dead surface cells can be removed. So be sure to reheat the tea from time to time as necessary, and continue the facial fomentations for 15 minutes. (Don't shorten the 15-minute time period as you won't get the same beneficial results.)

This treatment is completely safe to use and even helps to clear up certain skin disorders. The secret of its effectiveness lies in the papaya *enzymes* which actually dissolve the lifeless skin debris that prevents the living layers beneath from breathing. This formula will help maintain normal skin resiliency and tone which are fundamental to a youthful, soft complexion.

Almond Meal Cleanser

1. Almond meal is another successful herbal beauty aid for cleansing the skin, and is especially good for reducing oversized pores. Mix the almond meal with just enough water to make it creamy and spread this on your neck and face. Allow the mask to dry, and after ten or 15 minutes wash it off with gentle friction to loosen the dead skin particles. Used every day it helps to prevent or clear away blackheads, reduce enlarged pores, and freshen the skin.

2. Here is a quicky method of using the almond powder for skin cleansing: Pour a little of the powder into your hands with enough water to make it spread easily and use it just as you would soap to wash your face and hands. Rinse immediately.

Oatmeal Cleanser

Ordinary oatmeal is an old-time skin debris remover that still works wonders.

Mix uncooked oatmeal with buttermilk and smear this on your face. Let it dry and leave it on for 15 minutes to one-half hour. Then rinse, and blot the skin with a clean facial tissue or towel.

Peppermint Steam Facial

This is used only for oily or normal skin complexions.

A peppermint steam facial is a deep, deep cleanser. In the privacy of your own home you can enjoy the soothing action of warm herbal steam on your face. The fragrant mist opens pores to allow complete, thorough cleansing and also relaxes facial tensions. Just a few treatments and you'll find your skin glows with radiance and charm.

Directions: Place a handful of peppermint leaves in a large bowl and pour boiling water over them. Arrange a towel over your head as you hold your face over the steaming basin so that the swirling mist can be concentrated on the facial areas. Use for ten minutes. (Repeat as necessary.)

MAGIC FACIAL BEAUTY MASK

You don't need to spend your hard-earned money on expensive rare cosmetics to give your skin the look of radiant beauty. For only a few pennies a day and a few minutes of your time you can prepare a secret beauty treatment that will help erase the mask of age and add a natural glow and fine youthfulness to your complexion. This simple home-preparation is remarkably effective. Some famous movie stars who look ten or 20 years younger than their actual age have used this recipe to make time stand still for their skin.

For this youthifying process you will need:

> 1 bottle of pure olive oil
> 1 bottle of witch hazel (Keep refrigerated)
> 1 bottle of milk of magnesia
> 1 bar mild antiseptic soap

Directions: Use this treatment once a week.

First Step: Wash the face and neck thoroughly with mild antiseptic soap and warm water, then blot the skin dry with an absorbent towel.

Second Step: Shake the bottle of magnesia briskly and spread the liquid liberally over the face and neck. Leave it on the skin for several minutes until it has dried thoroughly. This milk of magnesia pack clears clogged pores and draws impurities from the skin.

Third Step: Now dissolve the dried mask by applying a second layer of magnesia directly over it, then remove with a warm damp towel.

Fourth Step: Heat a little olive oil to above body temperature and apply the oil gently with the finger tips to the cheeks, forehead, and neck, sweeping it into the skin in upward strokes. Allow the oil to remain for five minutes so that its deep moisturizing power can penetrate your tissues and help smooth away skin dryness and resulting lines, adding a flush of natural beauty to your complexion.

Final Step: When the five minutes are up, remove the excess olive oil by applying ice cold witch hazel with a small dab of cotton. The witch hazel also acts as an astringent, leaving your skin young, fresher, and firmer.

The Need to Be Patient

You may not notice much difference after the first or second treatment for during this time the process will be working to remove the build-up of grime from the pores. Once this is done the skin will respond, and after only three or four treatments your complexion will begin to take on a superb velvety smoothness and radiance. Crow's-feet around the eyes, wrinkles on the forehead and neck will begin to disappear. Even the contours of your face and neck will start to take on a more youthful line. You have to experience this treatment personally to convince yourself of its marvelous results.

Don't Forget Your Hands

Hands with skin that looks old can spoil your whole image, so after you have used the magic formula on your face and neck apply it to your hands. The result will be a more youthful firmness and lovelier skin texture—a real pleasure to behold.

THE BODY BEAUTIFUL

The following formula will stimulate the circulation, smooth the skin and help keep the body beautiful:

Mix:

6 oz. peanut oil
2 oz. olive oil
1 tsp. lanolin

Bottle for use.

This solution should be applied directly after a tepid bath in which the body has been thoroughly washed with castile soap.

Shake the bottle well before using. Begin by massaging the lotion on the face, neck, shoulders, and arms. Then go over the entire body, especially the limbs, abdomen, and diaphragm.

BEAUTY AIDS FOR SPECIFIC SKIN PROBLEMS

Pale Complexion—Greasy Skin

Parsley tea can be used effectively for pale complexions that need stimulation and toning, and as a rinse for greasy skin it is excellent.

Bring one pint of water to a boil. As soon as the water boils add a good handful of parsley and remove the pot from the burner immediately (continued boiling destroys the herb's valuable properties). Keep the parsley tea covered and allow it to steep for ½ hour. When the solution has cooled sufficiently, strain off the herb and rinse your face with the tea several times a day. This must be prepared fresh daily.

Blackheads—Blemishes—Enlarged Pores

1. This formula, used once a week, will do wonders for reducing enlarged pores and for clearing away blackheads and skin blemishes:

Remove the yolk from a raw egg and beat the *egg-white* until stiff, then mix this with one teaspoonful of honey. Smooth the mixture over the face with a pad of cotton or with your fingers. Leave it on for 15 minutes, then rinse with warm followed by cool water. Blot the face dry.

2. The following recipe is centuries old and is still a favorite among many people in different countries throughout the world. It is prepared and used the same as the previous formula:

Combine 3 ounces of ground barley with one ounce of honey and enough beaten egg-white to make a paste.

3. Here is a specific for blackheads:

Combine 8 oz. powdered almond meal, 4 oz. powdered orris root, 1 oz. powdered castile soap. Mix enough hot water with about one tablespoonful of the powder to form a paste. Spread this gently on the skin, and rub into the blackhead areas. Repeat the process several times until you feel that your skin has been thoroughly cleansed. Then rinse well with cold water.

Oily Skin

1. For oily skin, mix three ounces of cucumber juice with three ounces of witch hazel and 1½ ounces of rose water. Rub this into your skin with pads of cotton or use your finger tips. This cucumber lotion brings freshness and new breathing ability to the skin.

(To extract the cucumber juice, wash the cucumber, then grate it and squeeze through a cloth.)

2. A facial of yarrow flower tea is superb for greasy or oily skin conditions. Some herbalists recommend it for acne.

Put an ounce of dried or fresh yarrow flowers in a bowl and pour a pint of boiling water over them. Cover the bowl with a saucer and allow the infusion to steep (stand) for about ten minutes, then strain. Wring a cloth out loosely in the herb solution and hold the cloth on your face. As the cloth begins to lose its heat dip it into the tea and apply again. Reheat the liquid as necessary, as the compresses must be kept as hot as comfortably possible. Continue the hot fomentations for ten minutes, then pat the face dry without rinsing.

This process should be done twice a day, morning and evening. For best results, especially in conditions of acne, the procedure should be followed for several weeks.

3. Sage tea, prepared as ordinary tea, is a simple yet effective treatment for oily skin. Rinse your face with the strained solution several times a day.

4. For oily nose, mix one teaspoon of boric acid with four ounces of rose water. Apply this lotion on the nose as often as necessary.

Very Dry Skin

The USSR Institute of Medical Cosmetics offers the following for very dry skin conditions: The face should not be washed with soap and water. Instead, cleansing should be done with warm vegetable oil applied with cotton pads every evening.

Dry Itchy Skin

Fill a cloth bag with one pound of oatmeal and tie the bag securely. Place this right in your bath water. Relax in the tub and massage the skin gently with the oatmeal bag for about 20 minutes.

Dry or Scaly Skin

Here is a time-tested herbal aid for dry or scaly skin: Mix two teaspoonfuls of fine oatmeal with enough olive oil to form a soft paste. Add one-half cup of hot water. When cool, strain the mixture through muslin, squeezing thoroughly to extract the liquid. Dab the strained solution on the skin two or three times a day and allow it to soak in. This recipe must be prepared fresh at least every other day as it will not keep.

Freckles

1. Lemon juice is an old-time favorite for bleaching freckles. Apply to the freckled area and let it dry. Repeat every day until results are achieved.

2. Burdock prepared as a tea with distilled water makes an effective lotion for freckles and skin blemishes.

3. *Old Parisian Freckle Lotion:* Mix one ounce of lemon juice, one ounce of powdered alum, one pint of rose water. Place in a tightly capped bottle. Shake well and apply as necessary.

Stretch Marks—Converging Lines

Massage cocoa butter on areas where stretch marks or converging lines are visible, as between the eyebrows and around the mouth. This helps to soften the texture of the skin.

Chapped Hands

1. Add one ounce of rose water to one ounce of glycerine and one-half ounce of witch hazel. Shake well and apply to the hands as necessary.

As a preventive measure against chapping, use the lotion on your hands directly after they have been in water. Dry the hands thoroughly before using the solution.

2. Another aid for chapped hands is the use of sesame seed oil or almond oil as a lotion.

Chilblains

Applications of lemon juice mixed with glycerine is excellent for treating chilblains.

Calluses—Brittle Nails—Skin Cracks

Castor oil applied frequently to calluses will soften them. Olive oil also has a soothing effect on the skin. Rub the oil well into the hands at bedtime. It can also be applied to nails that show signs of splitting or brittleness.

For skin cracks on the fingers, apply sunflower seed oil frequently.

Rough Elbows and Knees

Massage almond oil into the areas several times a day.

If the rough elbows and knees are also discolored, rub them with half a lemon, then soak the parts with warm almond oil for ten minutes. This should be used once or twice a week. The result is smooth white knees and elbows once again.

Brown Spots

The appearance of brown spots on the hands and face is a cosmetic problem that generally affects men and women of mature years.

Different methods for removing these tell-tale aging signs have been used by many people. An old-time favorite remedy is castor oil rubbed into the brown spots every night until they disappear. Some sources recommend external applications of the fresh juice from ground-up parsley.

Modern authorities suggest supplementing the diet with vitamins C and E. Nutritionalist Adelle Davis advises taking 100 units of vitamin E after each meal.

Acne

Perhaps no skin disease causes as much social distress as acne. Cleanliness and correct nutrition are extremely important in preventing or treating this unpleasant skin disorder. Diets excessively high in fat content (cakes, candy, ice cream, fried foods, etc.) stimulate the sebaceous glands and the increased activity forces oils to the surface where they are sometimes clogged. The result is a pimple.

According to the *Journal of the American Medical Association*[1] a diet extremely low in fat might be helpful in skin problems of this type.

And there are other angles to treating or preventing acne. The anti-acne effects of vitamin A taken orally have been known for a long time. Recently, however, experiments over several years have shown that a solution containing vitamin A *acid* is more than twice as effective. (It is expected to be available soon by prescription.) In most cases experiments have demonstrated that the solution applied topically begins to clear up acne in three to five weeks and the skin is almost back to normal within three months. Penn researchers who made the important discovery were awarded a silver medal for Research in Skin Disease by fellow dermatologists.

---

[1] April 12, 1958.

How Medical Herbalists
Treat Acne and Other Skin Disorders

In addition to advocating a correct diet and cleanliness, medical herbalists prescribe various herbal formulas for the treatment of acne. For example, some herbalists recommend drinking cups of yarrow tea daily, along with hot fomentations (compresses) of a yarrow tea solution to the face. The tea as a beverage is prepared the same as ordinary tea. For external applications, the same formula given earlier in this chapter for yarrow and oily skin is used. For best results, medical herbalists advise that *both* the yarrow beverage and the hot fomentations of yarrow tea be employed for several weeks.

According to a journal of organic medicine, impressive results have been obtained with a herbal formula in the treatment of skin diseases such as acne, eczema, impetigo, boils, and dermatoses of untraceable origin. The journal states:[2]

> These complaints are well covered by the following: red clover flowers, two oz.; burdock root, one oz.; blue flag root, one oz.; sassafras bark, one-half oz.
>
> *Method:* Place one-quarter of the mixture in one pint of cold water, bring to the boil, simmer for 20 minutes, strain when cold.
>
> *Dose:* One wineglassful three times daily, until improvement is apparent.

Eczema

Researchers have reported many cases where unsaturated fatty acids added to the diet greatly improved conditions of eczema. (Any oil from a cereal or vegetable source contains these important unsaturated fatty acids; wheat germ, corn, sunflower seed, and safflower oils are examples.) The oils were used in cooking or given by the tablespoonful.

According to a report by the Lee Foundation,[3] 87 chronic cases of eczema responded to treatment with corn oils, though standard treatment employed for years had failed.

---

[2]*Health from Herbs,* February 1955.

[3]February 1942.

Psoriasis

The unsaturated fatty acids have also been found to have a beneficial effect on psoriasis. Tests among patients suffering from this skin disorder showed a low level of unsaturated fatty acids in the blood. When the oils were added to the diet, there was a prompt reduction in the skin disease.[4]

OTHER HERBAL BEAUTY AND GLAMOUR AIDS

For your "Sun-Day" Best

The sun is important to the health, but heavy doses can drain natural oils and moisture from the body and thereby hasten the skin-aging process. Overexposure to the sun's rays explains the dry leathery faces of many ranchers, farmers, and seamen.

Between the hours of 11 A.M. and 3 P.M. you get the burning infrared rays, which cause a breakdown in the body's tissues. If a person is in a toxic condition these harmful rays may even produce skin cancer.

There is no need to fear the sun if precautions are taken. If you spend a great deal of time outdoors, plan your hours to avoid heavy, intense sunlight, or make it a practice to wear a wide-brimmed hat and long sleeves. The best time for sunbathing is *before* 11 A.M. and *after* 3 P.M. Do your gardening early in the morning, then again in late afternoon and early evening. Rub a little cocoa butter on your hands, neck, and face before going out in the sun. This non-greasy beauty aid helps the skin to retain its moisture and to remain smooth and soft.

Quick Tanning Lotion

Here is a lotion you can prepare that hastens the tanning process and beneficially reduces the time you must expose your body to the sun.

Beat the yolk of an egg thoroughly, then slowly whip in one cup of olive or corn oil until the mixture thickens. Now add one tablespoon each of vinegar and wheat germ oil. Beat the entire

---

[4]*Archives of Research*, August 1954.

mixture together thoroughly and apply this to all parts of the exposed areas of your body before sunbathing.

Note: If you prefer to buy your own tanning creams already prepared, try those made of aloe vera. Aloe vera, a cactus-like desert plant, was prized by the lovely women of ancient Egypt and Greece for its remarkable beautifying effects. Suntan creams made from aloe vera and without the addition of synthetics help you attain a rich glowing tan while moisturizing and shielding your skin. Most health food stores carry these products.

Sunburn Lotion

Mix together one-half ounce each of olive oil, glycerine, and distilled witch hazel. Apply as required for the relief of sunburn.

For the Tender Skin of the Gums and Mouth

1. *Exotic Mouthwash and Breath Sweetener.* Mystic gum-myrrh was an ingredient used by the ancient Jews for anointing the holy Ark, the Tabernacle, the altars and the sacred vessels.

In modern times this ancient aromatic is employed to flavor wines, but its main use is in mouthwashes, dentifrices, perfumery and incense.

An excellent breath sweetener and mouthwash can be made simply by adding a little tincture of myrrh to a glass of water.

2. *Myrrh Dentifrice for the Smile of Sparkling Beauty.* To clean the teeth and gums, take one ounce of finely powdered myrrh, two teaspoonfuls of the best quality honey, and a little green sage in fine powder. Mix well together and rub the teeth and gums with a little of this balsam every night and morning. It also makes a wonderful breath sweetener as well as a dentifrice.

Nature's Deodorant

If you have carefully considered all the facts relating to the duties and functions of your skin you will realize that using a commercial underarm deodorant to keep you "dry" cannot possibly be healthful. Such preparations close off the pores and as a result prevent the excess water, salt, and toxins from escaping.

The storehouse of nature can supply you with an excellent

underarm deodorant that is both safe and 100% effective. Just use plain ordinary apple cider vinegar applied to the underarm area directly after bathing. Don't worry about the strong vinegar aroma for it quickly fades a few moments after it has been applied. This simple, inexpensive natural deodorant will keep you protected for many hours. It does not stop normal discharge of perspiration, but thoroughly eliminates the disagreeable underarm odor.

If you wish, the vinegar may be scented with fragrant herbs merely by steeping. Among some of the best botanicals for this purpose are rosemary, lavender flowers, marjoram, and orris root. Make your own blend or use a single botanical.

To prepare, simply bring a pint of apple cider vinegar to a boil, then add one ounce of the herb or herbs and turn off the burner immediately. Cover the container and allow the solution to steep (stand) until cold. Strain and bottle for use.

CHAPTER SUMMARY

1. Home preparations utilizing select herbs and natural foods as beauty aids can help your skin look more youthful and vibrant at only a fraction of the cost of expensive cosmetics.
2. Many commercial cosmetics contain antibiotics, hormones, or other irritants. By contrast, herbs used in do-it-yourself beauty recipes are harmless, with no side-effects.
3. Old-looking hands can spoil your whole image. Apply the appropriate herbal formulas in this chapter to your hands as well as to your face and neck for a more youthful appearance.
4. Do not prepare your herbal beauty aids in aluminum containers. Use containers lined with enamel, or made of Pyrex, glass, or household china.

13

Secrets of Longevity
Using Selected Herbs

Many scientists are now pooling their knowledge about aging and believe that a longer, more useful life is in our future. According to various studies it is believed that by the year 2000 we should all be living to be at least 100 years old, and perhaps more.

Discoveries in molecular biology have brought about a clearer understanding of the aging process. Scientists agree that these provide, in theory, a means of slowing down or even possibly halting the aging process. The implications of such a development are claimed to be of staggering importance.

One doctor in Mexico, specializing in biochemistry, predicted as many as 200 candles on future birthday cakes. In addressing a meeting of the Mexican Academy of Surgery, Dr. Manuel Mateos Fournier said that in view of the progress medicine has made, there is no reason why eventually humans should not live to be up to 200 years of age. He announced that chemicals to slow down the aging process are in various early stages of development, and "the possibility of a very long life for people, with complete possession of all their faculties, can be looked for within the very near future."

In the meantime a surprising number of people have already stretched their life span far beyond the proverbial threescore and ten by using their own personal do-it-yourself methods. Recent surveys show that over 13,000 living Americans have reached the magic age of 100 and over. Other countries have also reported thousands of cases in which people are living to a ripe old age.

THE LIFE STYLE OF THE OLDSTERS

A number of studies have been conducted on the life habits of people in the "100 plus" group. Essentially, the common outstanding traits shared by the majority were found to be: Adequate rest—retiring to bed early and rising early, plus a short nap or rest in the middle of the day; freedom from tension, stress, and worry; daily out-of-door exercise—walking in particular; regularity of daily habits; moderation in all things; a generally placid yet energetic disposition.

The majority did not drink or smoke. Most lived in their own homes or in some other independent situation. The proportion of those who came from long-lived families were about equal to those who did not. (One study of 27,181 Russians over the age of 80 found they had no more or no less long-lived ancestors than did the general population.) Obesity with its death-dealing side-effects was not found. Large meals were not eaten—eating little, but more frequently, was generally the rule followed. The majority particularly stressed the importance of keeping active both in mind and body, and were found to have many interests. It is also significant that they firmly believed in work and were active either at a paid job, household chores, or volunteer work. In their opinion, to remain inactive by giving yourself the excuse that you're too old to do much of anything is fatal.

Along with these traits, a number of the oldsters also mentioned an additional factor or factors (these varied greatly) which they personally believed contributed to their longevity. Of particular interest to us are those cases in which the use of herbs was cited.

HERBS—HEALTH BUILDERS AND AIDS TO LONGEVITY

Disease is one of the principal causes of premature aging and a short life span. A list of some 90 diseases was submitted to a number of prominent physicians, along with a request to indicate the percentage of deaths from those diseases which could have been prevented. Calculations on the basis of returns indicated that through a possible timely prevention, more than a dozen years could have been added to life!

Diseases of the circulatory system of heart, arteries, and kidneys, generally due to atherosclerosis, called the "true killer," takes the greatest toll of life after the age of 40. Between the ages of 70 and 80 atherosclerosis accounts for two-thirds of all deaths.

Efforts to lengthen our years on earth must therefore be directed first to the prevention of disease, especially that of the circulatory system. With this thought in mind, let us turn our attention to those cases in which the individual has cited the use of a particular herb or herbs as the additional factor(s) which he personally believes has contributed greatly to his longevity.

You will note as we go along that in some of these cases the herb mentioned not only proves to be an important disease preventive and healing agent of certain conditions, but that it also has an ancient reputation for dealing effectively with the ravages of time. Identical beliefs about a specific plant being a "longevity herb" have appeared in all parts of the world among races completely isolated from each other. It seems unlikely that even the earliest of men were so foolish as to sustain a belief century after century without some kind of evidence to support it. It may well be that certain herbs contain an unknown element conducive to longevity that has yet to be discovered by science.

GARLIC AND LONGEVITY

Several years ago a 104-year-old great-great-grandmother paid a visit to her old neighborhood in Manhattan's lower East side. According to news reports, she made the trip alone from the home of a granddaughter 72 miles away.

But here in the big city with its teaming millions the centenarian found that crooks are no respecters of old age. She showed up at police headquarters to report the theft of her purse, which contained $20 and her railroad ticket home.

The police took the old lady to a city shelter and the next morning turned her over to a welfare caseworker. After some questioning, the caseworker located the granddaughter, who soon arrived to take grandma home.

Before leaving, the aged woman decided to pass along a longevity tip to her police befrienders. She advised that twice a day they take a teaspoon of crushed garlic and vodka. "The garlic brings the blood pressure down," she said, "and the vodka helps the circulation."

Garlic's Reputation As Longevity Herb

The reputation of garlic as a longevity and medicine herb can be traced back to the earliest times. This ancient folk-remedy was prescribed by the Egyptian priest-physicians over 5000 years ago, and its use is also mentioned in the ancient writings of the Chinese, Greeks, Romans, and Babylonians.

Throughout the long history of folk-medicine one finds innumerable references to the use of garlic for treating an infinite variety of ailments, but it was not until the 20th century that medical science finally began to take an interest in garlic as a possible therapeutic agent.

Electrobiologist Lauds Garlic

Some time ago Professor G. Tallarico wrote: "Lakhovsky [an electrobiologist] relates marvels of garlic and the onions because of their content of elements and specific essences. He says that in certain forests of Siberia a variety of wild garlic grows, called locally 'ceremissa.' Every autumn there is a pilgrimage to those forests when the aged, the paralysed, the sick, and those afflicted with all kinds of disease repair there to eat of the wild garlic for days, or even weeks. Afterward they return to their homes relieved of their ills, rejuvenated and healed. It is further said that in Russia and Poland there are groups of very pious and very poor Israelities who from time to time interrupt their religious exercises to break their fast upon bread and raw garlic. Cancer is unknown among those people, whose life span averages better than a century."

Doctor Praises Garlic

Kristine Nolfi, M.D., mentions that in both Yugoslavia and Bulgaria garlic is used in the average household almost every day. She draws attention to the fact that in these countries many individuals are over 100 years of age and still able to put in a full day's work.

Dr. Nolfi cites many of the healing virtues of garlic. For example: "Garlic has a strengthening and laxative effect, lowers too-high blood pressure and raises one which is too low; it also cures indigestion, disinfects the contents of the stomach of those who lack hydrochloric acid in their gastric juice for this purpose, kills putrefaction bacteria in the large intestines, and neutralizes poisons in the organism itself."

The Famed Abkhasians—Garlic Users

Much has been written about the Abkhasians, remarkably long-lived people of the Caucasus. One researcher found that 40 percent of the men and 30 percent of the women in a group of Abkhasians over the age of 90 could see well enough to thread a needle without glasses. In another instance, doctors obtained sperm from one man who was 119!

In the articles about the life style and habits of these long-lived people we find that they practice an elaborate system of herbal folk medicine, and among the foods mentioned in their diets, "large quantities of garlic are always on hand."

Anti-bacterial Powers

One of the known ingredients responsible for the power of garlic as an anti-infection agent is *allinin*. Wallace E. Harrel, M.D., reported that he found *allinin* inhibited growth in large numbers of Gram-positive and Gram-negative microbes. Other scientists have also recognized the anti-bacterial power of garlic.

Anti-tumor Activities Studied

Prolonged experiments at the Kyoto University in Japan demonstrated that when tumor cells are treated with garlic extract and then injected into mice, the mice developed a strong immunity to the same type of tumor cells. Drs. Natata and Fugiwara found that only the extract of fresh garlic brought about the immunity. If the garlic was boiled first, it did not protect the mice and the tiny creatures died in two to four weeks. By contrast, during an observation period of ten weeks none of the fresh garlic-tumor injected mice died.

The power of garlic against cancer in mice was also reported in a scientific journal, where F. Kroning stated that "there exists a complete inhibition of the mammary-tumors in the female C_3H-mice by fresh garlic."

A Life-long Protector Against a Host of Ailments

Dr. Madaus of Germany demonstrated that garlic relieves nicotine poisoning.

Other scientific researchers have found that the little garlic bulb is remarkably effective in preventing tuberculosis, pneumonia, diphtheria, and typhus; that it is useful in all respiratory infections, especially in symptoms of dry hacking coughs, in colds, asthma, and bronchitis; that it relieves dyspepsia, colic, and flatulence, and is an excellent nerve tonic. Further, that it kills round and thread body worms, and is a good remedy for certain cases of dysentery or diarrhoea; also it is a counter-irritant and rubefacient which may be used with advantage in compress form for pleurisy, tuberculosis of the larynx, intercostal neuralgia and catarrhal pneumonia.[1]

Don't Delay—Do It Now!

There is no need to wait until you are ill, when you can help prevent disease by adding as much fresh garlic to your meals as possible. Garlic can be included in almost any meat, cheese, egg, or vegetable dish, and can be added to all soups and salads. If you don't care for the taste of garlic, or if you are concerned about the odor it leaves on your breath, the answer to your problem is to take garlic perles. These natural concentrates of garlic do not dissolve until they are far down in your digestive system.

ONION AND LONGEVITY

According to various reports, Zora Agha of Turkey lived to the age of 142. It was said that he ate only one meal a day, which consisted chiefly of black bread and onions. Dr. Edmund Szekely

---

[1]*New York Physician,* September 1937.

tells us that when Agha was 140 years of age, an enterprising American business man took him on an exhibition tour in the United States. Unfortunately the dramatic switch from his life-long diet to two years of eating meat in restaurants proved too much for the old man and brought about his demise.

A Potent Germ Killer

The onion belongs to the same herb family as garlic, and has been used for centuries for treating a wide variety of ailments ranging from circulatory disorders to the common cold. Today, most Europeans still regard onions and garlic as near panaceas (cure-alls).

The action of onions in lung disease and on the mucous lining of the nose and throat is well known. Modern research, both in our own country and abroad, has shown that the unassuming bulb is a potent germ killer. Chewing on an onion for five minutes destroys all harmful bacteria in the lining of the mouth.

Soviet medical investigators reported that they have successfully treated severely infected open wounds with applications of onion poultices.

Medical Marvel in Onions

The medical profession has taken considerable interest in the therapeutic possibilities of onions for treating high blood pressure and other problems of the circulatory system. For example, a team of British doctors has demonstrated with tests on humans that onions boiled or fried can help reduce the possibility of heart attacks by raising the blood's capacity to dissolve or prevent deadly internal clots. (In the tests, convalescent patients were given a portion of onions along with their breakfast or lunch.)

The doctors go on to say that there are drugs which will prevent excessive clotting, but these are very expensive, transient in effect, or have an unwanted side effect. Pharmaceutical firms are now busy searching for the basic ingredient in onions that may lead to the development of a cheaper, non-harmful medication.

Aid to Solo Voyager

A few years ago, *Prevention* magazine[2] cited the story of Wilfried Erdmann, a 27-year-old German carpenter who astonished authorities when he returned in perfect health from the ordeal of a solo sailing trip of 20 months. Unlike most world voyagers emerging from similar trips, his bodily vitamin stores were not depleted and his skin did not suffer from sun and salt. Erdmann attributed his remarkable condition to the 100 pounds of onions he took with him on his trip.

Beneficial Ultraviolet Radiation of Onions

Some time ago, Professor Gurwitch announced that a peculiar type of ultraviolet radiation was emitted by onions. These radiations, called M-rays, appeared to stimulate cell activity and produce a rejuvenating effect on the system. Garlic and ginseng[3] were also found to emit the same radiation.

The Answer to Many Health Problems

In view of scientific research on the humble onion it appears that the bulb may be the answer to many of our health problems. The onion is a food, obviously a very important food, and could be eaten along with garlic every day for maximum results.

CAYENNE AND LONGEVITY

At the age of 110, Mr. George Gibbs of Walla Walla, Washington, was still doing his own household chores and cutting his own firewood. Over the past ten years he has had various honors bestowed on him, his most highly prized being a congratulatory letter he received near his 102nd birthday from President John F. Kennedy.

In his long life, Gibbs has seen a great many changes. For instance, he was four years old when Abraham Lincoln was

---

[2]May 1969.

[3]Information on ginseng as a rejuvenation herb has been fully covered in my book, *Nature's Medicines* (Parker Publishing Company, West Nyack, New York 10994).

assassinated, 15 when Bell invented the telephone, and 42 when the Wright brothers made aviation history.

At the time of this writing, Gibbs is nearing his 111th birthday. He possesses a fine sense of humor and enjoys greeting his visitors with a series of wisecracks. In view of his remarkable age, his memory is astonishingly good.

Mr. Gibbs attributes his longevity to large daily doses of cayenne pepper which he says he takes "right from the spoon." He claims that his father lived to be 100 and also used cayenne regularly.

Varied Opinions

Anyone who has followed the history of folk medicine finds that cayenne is occasionally cited as a longevity herb, and always as a powerful stimulant and important remedy for treating various forms of illness. For medicinal purposes it was generally used in the form of a tea, and in recent years either as a tea, or placed in capsules and swallowed with a glass of water. But to what extent and how regularly doses of cayenne pepper may be safely taken by a healthy person is a controversial matter. Some claim that its constant use, even in fairly large amounts, is perfectly harmless, and to back up their argument point to people of tropical lands such as Mexico where the herb is used freely as a condiment in hot sauces and food dishes. However, in these cases the herb is not used alone.

Others state that cayenne taken by itself should be used carefully and with the utmost discretion. For example, a medical herbalist who employed cayenne in his practice expressed his own opinion and that of many of his colleagues when he wrote: "In advocating the use of cayenne we do not wish to be understood that it will cure everything, nor do we recommend it to be taken regularly, whether a stimulant is required or not."

Until further scientific research has been done with this herb, no one should take daily doses of cayenne pepper such as Mr. Gibbs has been doing all his life. However, since cayenne is occasionally listed among the longevity herbs in the archives of folk medicine, in all fairness let us take a closer look at this plant to which Mr. Gibbs attributes his extreme age.

The Properties of Cayenne

Cayenne (*Capsicum*) is a large genus of tropical shrubs having small flowers succeeded by dry, many-seeded brown berries called chilies or peppers. The word *capsicum* is taken from the Greek *kapto* "I bite," in allusion to the herb's hot, biting taste. Paprika is the milder pungent spice of the many varieties, and is known botanically as *Capsicum tetragonum*. The chief kinds are *Hungarian paprika*, made from the pods only, after removal of the stalks and seeds, and *king's paprika*, where pods, seeds, and stalks are used.

Paprika Contains Vitamin C and Potassium

The people of Hungary have used paprika liberally on their food for centuries and are thoroughly convinced that it has been a valuable contributing factor to their good health and temperament. When Professor Szent-Gyorgyi, the discoverer of vitamin C, returned to Hungary from the United States after his unsuccessful attempts to produce this valuable vitamin from tons of liver, he accidently found that red pepper is an exceptionally rich source of vitamin C. (It also contains a high amount of potassium.)

Past Uses in Fevers and Battle Fatigue

Cayenne pepper, the hot pungent spice commonly called "capsicum," is made from the fruit of several species, chiefly from *Capsicum annum* and *Capsicum frutescens*.

The inhabitants of tropical climates employ capsicum as a remedy for various ailments. Dr. Watkins, for example, reported that when sick with fever, the natives of the West Indies drink freely of a tea made by steeping cayenne pods in hot water to which sugar and the juice of oranges is added.

In his *Pharmacologica*, Paris wrote that French army surgeons prescribed cayenne for soldiers who were battle weary and fatigued.

Recorded Uses in Various Ailments

Cayenne was frequently administered by the old-time family physicians and was a particular favorite of the Thomsonian System of Botanic Medicine. Other practitioners of herbal remedies also valued the herb. Here are a few excerpts from the writings of those times:

"In all diseases prostrating in their nature ... capsicum is invaluable in the prescription as the toning agent which helps the system throw off the disease and reestablish equilibrium."

"There are many languid people who need something to make the fire of life burn more brightly. Capsicum, not whiskey, is the thing to do it."

"In chronic and sluggish conditions, the small dose [of cayenne] frequently given is 1 to 3 grains with either hot or cold water."

"It [cayenne] has a pungent taste, which continues for a considerable length of time; when taken into the stomach it produces a pleasant sensation of warmth, which soon diffuses itself throughout the whole system, equalizing the circulation. Hence it is so useful in inflammation and all diseases which depend upon a morbid increase of blood in any particular part of the body."

"In colds, relaxed throat, cold condition of the stomach, dyspepsia, spasms, palpitation, particularly in the acute stages, give a warm infusion [tea] of capsicum in small repeat doses, about two teaspoonfuls every half hour or more frequently if required."

"The African bird pepper [cayenne] is the purest and the best stimulant known. It has a pungent taste, and is the most persistent heart stimulant ever known. It is exceedingly prompt in its effects. Through the circulation, its influence is manifest through the whole body. The heart first, next the arteries, then the capillaries, and the nerves."

CAYENNE IN MODERN USE

Capsicum still holds an important place in the materia medica of the modern herbal practitioner. It also enters into the manufacture of many liniments and ointments which are sold in drug stores.

A recent volume of the *U. S. Dispensatory* gives this information on the internal use of cayenne:

Capsicum is a powerful local stimulant, producing, when swallowed, a sense of heat in the stomach, and a general glow over the body without any narcotic effect. It is much employed as a condiment, especially in hot climates, and may be useful in cases of atony of the stomach and intestines. It is contraindicated in cases of gastric inflammation, though in the chronically inflamed stomachs of persons of intemperate habits it frequently appears to do good. It may also be of value in certain cases of serous diarrhoea, not dependent on true inflammation of the intestines.

C. F. Leyel writes: "Capsicum helps the feeble digestion of those addicted to alcohol, who suffer from a loss of vitality and a sluggish condition. When taken internally, it is a powerful stimulant; it promotes digestion and cures flatulence. It makes a good gargle. . . . It is a good remedy for nasal catarrh."

A recent issue of a periodical on botanic medicine lists cayenne as follows:

CAYENNE

Synonyms: African pepper, Bird pepper, Red pepper, Capsicum.

Action: Stimulant, tonic, carminative, diaphoretic, rubefacient.

Uses: One of the strongest and purest stimulants known. . . . A tonic for all organs of the body including the heart. Expels worms. . . . Sprinkled freely in socks against frostbite. Used for fumigation. Gives tone to the circulation. Said to increase fertility and delay senility. Persons exposed for any length of time to cold and damp may ward off disease by taking pills made from pure cayenne. A West Indian remedy for scarlatina. Wards off seasickness.

Domestic Use: Cayenne pepper is extremely hot and should be used sparingly. A small amount is a valuable addition in cheese dishes, sauces, egg dishes, and with shell fish.

(Note the remark in the above account that the herb is said to delay senility.)

THE LONGEVITY SECRETS OF G. E. D. DIAMOND

Goddard Ezekiel Dodge Diamond died 1916 at the advanced age of 120. The additional factors to which Diamond attributed his longevity were the drinking of distilled water in place of tap water, and the daily use of olive oil. He said, "Its [olive oil's] reconstructive properties follow the external application as readily as when given internally."

It was not until he was 40 years of age that Diamond experienced his first bout with illness, an attack of "black measles," the results of which impaired his vision and hearing. These effects he hoped would disappear with time but after three years there was still no improvement. He said, "my eyes were very painful, water running from them and a film gathering over them. My hearing was quite dull and growing worse."

His Experience with Olive Oil

At this point he recalled the deep interest he had had "in the reading of the Hebrew kings, how they were anointed with oil, and how oil was used as a means of healing and physical preservation." So Diamond decided to try the best oil he could possibly obtain for external application, and selected pure olive oil. This he applied to his eyes and eyelids, also beneath the eyes and under the eyelids. He claimed that after two or three applications the improvement was so pronounced that he decided to employ olive oil for his hearing as well. "I used the oil freely about the ears externally, and put drops of oil into the ears, holding it there with bits of cotton balls. In a very short time my sight and hearing were entirely restored."

The Oldster's Secret

When in his 60's, Diamond discovered symptoms of rigidity in his joints and bones. He said, "One day I jumped from a wagon to the ground and my joints did not respond with the usual rebound." Diamond, startled and surprised at this, promptly climbed back onto the wagon and jumped again. "The proof was there," he sadly acknowledged, "for not only did the knees refuse to rebound, but the backbone creaked and cried out in pain."

Diamond lost no time getting out his bottle of olive oil. He outlined the practice he followed of using the oil daily, sometimes both morning and evening for the remainder of his life: First he took a sponge bath with a wet soaped towel, "rubbing every part as thoroughly and as rapidly as possible." After rinsing, and drying himself with a coarse towel, he rubbed his body with a brush to further stimulate the circulation. Then pouring a little olive oil into the hollow of his hand he began applying it to his joints, "on the inside especially, that is, under the arms, in elbows, in rear of knees, on the insteps and in the groins." Next he rubbed the oil on his "shoulders, spine, hips, knees, bottoms of the feet, and frequently on top of the head."

Apparently the oil worked wonders for him as we are told by various writers that when Diamond was past the age of 100 he was doing gymnastics that few young men could equal; that at the age of 108 he was riding a bicycle and walking 20 miles a day; that sometimes he attended social events, and on one occasion, at the age of 110 he danced most of the evening with a young girl of 16.

Pure Virgin Olive Oil

Diamond also praised the internal use of olive oil, stating that in his opinion the oil "stands unrivaled as an element of natural food." He claimed that "one spoonful" three to five times a day on an empty stomach was excellent for stiff joints, indigestion, liver derangements, gall stones, stomach trouble, constipation, and many other ailments.

Diamond repeatedly stressed the importance of employing only the pure virgin olive oil whether it was to be used internally or externally. He pointed out that many cheaper varieties of olive oil are adulterated with cotton seed oil.

MODERN USES OF OLIVE OIL

Cholesterol

Scientific studies in France, Yugoslavia and elsewhere have shown that daily doses of olive oil can effectively reduce blood cholesterol.

Heart and Artery Diseases

On the Greek islands of Corfu and Crete, only four cases of heart and artery disease were found during a six-year study of

1,215 men between the ages of 40 and 59. The famous cardiologists who undertook the study reported at an international meeting of heart specialists in Athens that olive oil plays an important role in the diet of Greeks, and this factor appears related to their low mortality from heart disorder.

Stomach Ulcers

Dr. J. Dewitt Fox treated his ulcer patients with olive oil. He says: "Two tablespoons of olive oil with, or followed by, six ounces of milk do the same or even better a job of healing than the cream. It will also reduce the stomach acids, and because the oil is unsaturated will not raise the blood cholesterol."

Gallstones

Dr. E. Granata reports in an issue of *Minerva Dietologica* that he found olive oil to be a valuable preventive of gallstones.

Bursitis

One woman suffering from painful bursitis of her shoulder decided to try olive oil after reading of a case where the use of the oil had cleared up the painful condition. Every day she applied hot olive oil to her shoulder and upper arm, massaging and working the oil in gently but thoroughly. She began to improve, and gradually the movement came back to her shoulder. Before long she was able to raise her arm over her head. There have been no further attacks of bursitis since.

Cholesterol-Reducing Foot Bath

Another woman claimed that soaking her feet for ten minutes every day in a hot foot-bath prepared with shavings of castile soap reduced her blood cholesterol. She said, "I know it sounds crazy, but it worked—it really did! The drop in cholesterol was confirmed by my doctor." She went on to explain that she got the idea for using the footbath from a letter published in a magazine in which the writer wanted to pass the tip along to others.

Castile soap of course is made with pure olive oil.

Constipation

Modern medicine agrees with folk medicine that a dose of approximately one-half to two ounces of olive oil is a mild, effective laxative in chronic constipation. Some doctors also recommend its use in the form of an enema for fecal impactions.

Miscellaneous

Olive oil enters into the manufacture of cosmetics, toilet soaps, hair preparations, shampoos, skin lotions, liniments, and ointments.

HERBAL POLLEN FOR LONGEVITY

Inside the blossoms of herbs and flowers is a fine powder, usually yellow in color, which is commonly known as pollen.

In Norse mythology, the pagan gods were said to eat a secret food called *ambrosia,* which accounted for their immortality. Ambrosia was a combination of honey and bee bread, another name for the pollen stored in honeycomb cells. According to ancient texts of Babylon, Egypt, Persia, and China, it was agreed that this remarkable plant substance held the magic key to the secret of strength, health, and longevity.

Today the eating of pollen is still practiced in many regions of the world where ancient lore still survives. Island natives who live a more natural, primitive life, cherish pollen as a youth sustainer and valuable remedy for many ills. On certain islands of Hawaii, for example, natives use pollen from a type of pine (Pandanus plant) in the belief that it keeps them healthy and youthful.

According to reports, the natives of the Burma jungles remain energetic and vigorous right up to advanced years. They are tall, lean, and have perfect teeth. An important part of their daily diet is pollen honey-cakes; they also store some of the pollen in powdered form for medicinal purposes.

Pollen—Nature's Secret of Long Life?

Back in 1945 Nicolai Tsitsin, a Russian biologist, investigated ways of prolonging human life. Questionnaires were mailed to 200 people in Russia who claimed to be over 100 years of age. Of this number, 150 replied. Tsitsin wrote: "We made a very interesting discovery. The answers showed that a large number of them were bee keepers. But all of them without exception said that their principal food always had been honey." He then discovered that in each case "it wasn't really honey these people ate, but the waste matter in the bottom of the beehive." Tsitsin went on to explain that these people were all poor and sold the pure honey in the market, and kept only the residue for themselves. Further investigation revealed that a large part of this scrap honey was not honey but almost pure pollen.

Benefits of Using Pollen

During the years that followed, scientists in different countries began experiments with pollen, first on animals, and then on humans. Dr. Remy Chauvin of France reported increasing vitality and greater reproduction through several generations of mice fed exclusively on pollen for two years. Reporting on experiments in which pollen was administered to humans he said, "The first attempts at its use for symptoms of old age have proven most encouraging." He also found that pollen produced an increase of weight and strength during convalescence; that it brought about a rapid increase in the red blood cells of anemic children; and that it was effective against chronic constipation. In addition, he stated: "Interesting observations were registered in cases of flatulence as well as colonic infections. Patients suffering from chronic diarrhea which even resisted antibiotic treatment showed improvement." It was carefully noted that absolutely no ill effects were suffered by the many persons who took pollen regularly over a considerable length of time.

Cancer Research

Cancer researchers have experimented with feeding pollen to a strain of mice bred to develop tumors. Results showed that controlled amounts of pollen delayed the appearance of those tumors.

Valuable Constituents in Pollen

Two European universities agreed that hardly a foodstuff exists in either the vegetable or animal kingdom in which so many varied essentials of digestive needs are so completely united as in the case of pollen. They termed it one of the richest plant substances, even going so far as to say that it is "without equal in Nature."

An analysis by scientific researchers in Switzerland shows that pollen contains protein, free amino acids, various forms of sugar, mucilage, fats, minerals, trace elements, large quantities of the vitamin B complex, and also vitamins A, D, E, and C. "Uncounted diastase and hormone components, and antibiotics complete this already extraordinary versatile food. In addition there is no doubt that this product contains other active ingredients not yet known."

The Swiss researchers conclude by saying, "It is evident that pollen's content of elements important to life is extremely high. In many respects it exceeds the content of yeast, sprouted grain and royal jelly, which are known as being extremely vitalizing."

A Case History Involving Pollen

All the precious elements contained in pollen work together in a team effort to help you keep more youthful even when you are in your senior years. This was found to be true by many people. For example, a woman 73 years of age writes:

"About two years ago I began feeling terribly tired, draggy, no energy or pep—I had to drive myself to get my small amount of daily housework done. But what alarmed me was that my mind was getting confused and I also noticed signs of forgetfulness. I have seen many old people in such a senile state that they didn't even know their own children, and I was terribly afraid that this might eventually happen to me.

"On the suggestion of a friend, I thought I'd try pollen. I sent for a good supply and took three teaspoonfuls daily. Two weeks later the tiredness left me and I felt a remarkable surge of energy. I continued taking the pollen daily, and to my great joy, over a period of weeks my mental alertness gradually returned. No longer was there any confusion or lapses of memory. Today my mind is as sharp as it was in my younger years and I feel simply wonderful. Pollen will always be a part of my daily diet for the rest of my life."

   Note: Pollen taken by itself is quite bitter; therefore, where it has been widely consumed it is generally in combination with honey.

Commercially, it is sold in the form of pellets with enough honey to hold the powdery substance together. One to three teaspoonfuls may be taken daily.

THE CHINESE LONGEVITY HERB

The Chinese art of herbal healing has survived for thousands of years, during which time a great mass of herb remedies have accumulated. Therefore it is not surprising to find references to longevity herbs among the plants listed in the Chinese materia medica.

As stated in one of my previous books, the power to prolong life is among the virtues Orientals attribute to ginseng root. Although ginseng may be taken by both men and women, Chinese healers regard it primarily as a "man's herb" whereas the female equivalent of ginseng is a root called *Dong Kwei.*

Like ginseng, *Dong Kwei* has been used in China for ages. The Chinese claim it has remarkable powers for nourishing female glands, rebuilding blood, and helping to delay the symptoms of old age in women. If *Dong Kwei* does indeed nourish the female glands as the Orientals claim, we may have an important clue as to why it may qualify as a longevity herb.

In youth the female sex glands, like those of the male, are healthy and active. It is generally agreed that the vital hormones produced by healthy sex glands are directly related to the general health and to the prolonged appearance of youth. But with advancing age a gradual decline in the output of these hormones becomes evident. This decline usually begins in late middle years and is partly responsible for the symptoms of aging. When the sex glands are nourished, the precious hormones are once again produced at higher levels similar to those produced by younger people. In short, the new supply of hormones would help delay the symptoms of old age.

Case History

Mrs. P. W., a Chinese American, appears far younger than her chronological age of 84. She is in better shape physically, mentally, and psychologically than some people in their 50's or 60's. Mrs. P. W. does all her own shopping, cooking, and household chores, and still engages in her profession as a piano teacher which requires good mental discipline, memory, and agile movement of the arms, hands, and fingers. In addition, she participates in many social activities. When asked how she manages to remain so youthful, she opened her kitchen cabinet and held up a strange looking root. "This is *Dong Kwei,*" she said, "and I have used it ever since I was a young woman."

A Potent Herb

The stubby whitish-grey roots of *Dong Kwei* are usually from two to four inches long and have a very distinctive pungent odor. It is essential that these roots be stored in a dry place, otherwise they tend to soften and spoil. A good quality of *Dong Kwei* and the Chinese method used for preparing the herb results in a potent beverage. Therefore the Chinese women use it only once or twice a month. However, since the herb is also regarded as a blood builder, Chinese healers recommend that for conditions of anemia the herb broth should be taken more often until the blood becomes normal, and thereafter only once or twice a month (for nourishing the female glands).

Method of Preparation

Place four cups of water in a large Pyrex or enamelware container. Do not use aluminum; even stainless steel may not be used for this particular herb. Add a few pieces of lean raw chicken or beef and one small *Dong Kwei* root, or half of a large one. Cover loosely and bring to a boil. Reduce heat, then allow the herb broth to cook slowly for several hours or until the liquid is reduced to one and a half or two cups. Strain and drink the broth warm.

CHAPTER SUMMARY

1. Disease is one of the principal causes of aging and a short life span; consequently, efforts to lengthen our years must first be directed to the prevention of illness, especially that of the circulatory system.
2. Both the garlic and the onion contain medical marvels that may provide the answer to many of our health problems. Because of their remarkable power to heal or to prevent various ailments, these humble herbs of the lily family can increase our chances of living to a ripe old age.
3. Garlic should be eaten in as nearly the natural state as possible. Those who do not care for the taste of garlic or who find its odor objectionable may use garlic perles.
4. Researchers have found that pollen's content of elements important to life is extremely high and vitalizing. These precious elements work together in a team effort to help both body and mind remain more vigorous, healthy, and youthful, even in advanced age.
5. According to Chinese herbalists, the herb *Dong Kwei* has remarkable powers for nourishing the female glands, rebuilding blood, and helping to delay the symptoms of old age in women.
6. Case histories and various studies indicate that the process of "growing old" with the encroachment of certain degenerative conditions may be slowed down when the body is supplied with specific herbs or herb substances.

14

Herbal Glamorizers for Daily Use in the Home

In the social life of the ancient civilizations, aromatic herbs and pungent spices were the essence of personal luxury and an important part of public functions and private affairs. Perfumed smoke from scented candles and glowing sandalwood incense swirled through the royal chambers of mighty Oriental kings. Fragrant herb oils were placed in sacred temples for acceptance by the gods. The Arab women of Nubia burned cloves, ginger, cinnamon and other aromatics on a small charcoal fire to produce scented fumes for cleansing and perfuming their bodies. The Greeks and Romans filled their urns with spicy herbs to give their dwellings an enchanting fragrance. At some of his banquets Nero had sparkling fountains of rose water bubbling in the halls and garlands of rose blossoms placed around the necks of his guests.

The proverbial "bed of roses" is not entirely poetic fancy. Verres, a Roman politician, was in the habit of traveling on a litter padded with rose leaves, while the Sybarites used to sleep on mattresses stuffed with roses.

In the fabulous empire of the Pharoahs, caches of exotic frankincense and myrrh were buried in tombs with other treasures. Myrrh was an important ingredient in the famous Egyptian Kuphi, the oldest perfume known in man's history. Kuphi was the exquisite perfume Cleopatra used to charm her admirers, Mark Antony and Caesar. It was said that the sails of Cleopatra's ship were so heavily scented that the aroma heralded the ship's approach long before the vessel could be sighted.

Heaven-Scent

The Egyptians dispatched their own expeditions over the Red Sea to the Land of Punt (Land of God) for sweet-scented gums, barks, herbs, and spices. A remarkable record of such an expedition launched by the Egyptian Queen Hapshetsut has been preserved on the walls of the Queen's temple at Deir-el-Bahri. Detailed drawings and lengthy inscriptions reveal a fleet of five large galleys, each with 30 rowers, returning with a large cargo of "fragrant woods of God's land, heaps of myrrh-resin, of fresh myrrh trees . . . cinnamon wood, with incense, eye cosmetics . . . ."

Only the natural aromatics fresh from the hand of God could have produced the enchanting fragrance which appealed so strongly to these ancient people. Further emphasis of this fact is clearly shown in the following words from the Song of Harper written during the reign of King Antuf of the 11th dynasty:

> Immerse thyself in precious perfumes
> Which are the veritable products of the Gods.

The Questionable Safety of Synthetics

Unfortunately, most of our modern scented products are no longer composed solely of natural essences and oils. Synthetic chemicals have been added which we are sure would cause the ancient gods to hold their sacred noses at the sickeningly sweet odors wafting from aerosols and from various colognes, perfumes, hair sprays and toilet soaps that surround us on all sides. Nothing nature has created could possibly smell like that! And the number of chemical additives may or may not be harmful. Had you lived in grandmother's day, and used colognes, perfumes, sachets, and potpourri, there was no chance whatever that anything dangerous could result any more than if you carried a carnation in your lapel or a twig of rosemary in your pocket.

Artificial Odors Everywhere

To make matters worse, today we are exposed to many other sources of synthetic aromas. When housewives complained that wash dried in a drier did not come out smelling as fresh as clothes dried in the sunshine, manufacturers treated the driers with an invented odor to approximate the clean sunshine smell. Inner doors of refrigerators were smell-conditioned after it was found that certain plastics used in making the doors were causing off-odors and tastes in the foods. An aerosol containing the scent of new glue, solvents, and plastics has been made which can be sprayed into older cars to give the potential buyer the idea that he is getting something newer than it actually is.

Many lighter fluids, furniture polishes, candles, scouring powders and pads, paints, charcoal briquets, fly sprays, room deodorants, and toilet tissues are synthetically scented. As a result we are overwhelmed with cheap, imitation odors, and the effect on our lungs of breathing in droplets of moisture from chemical sprays and from the fumes rising from the concoctions we spread around our rooms cannot possibly be healthful.

NATURAL HOUSEHOLD DEODORIZERS

Back in the days when aerosols were unknown and houses were tightly shuttered against cold gloomy winter months, the natural aroma of plant substances were a "must" for anyone who had a sensitive nose. Stale musty smells and other objectionable household odors were completely overcome by fragrant botanicals. Nothing was more pleasant or refreshing.

Genuine aromatics are just as effective today as they were in olden times. They may be used to freshen up rooms for your own enjoyment and before guests arrive for social affairs. Or you can use them to mask cooking, smoking, or other unpleasant odors.

Fragrant Orange Deodorizer

1. Peel an orange and place a few of the peelings on the oven racks. Heat the oven to 350° and leave the oven door open. In a short while your whole house will be filled with the delightful woody fragrance of the orange peels. This simple method is also excellent for eliminating the peculiar odor resulting from some chemical oven cleaners.

2. Another way of permeating the atmosphere of your home with the charming orange aroma is simply to toss a few orange peels onto the lighted logs in your fireplace.

Mystic Fragrance

The incense-like aroma of rosemary is suggestive of ancient mystic rituals and ceremonies. You can perfume your home by burning a few dry sprigs of the herb in the fireplace. Or you can place them around the rooms, under shelf paper, on book cases, or on windowsills. The sprigs can be freshened up from time to time with a few drops of rosemary oil.

Another method is to prepare the herb as a decoction (a good handful to a quart of water). Reduce to a slow boil and leave the cover off. As the brew continues to simmer, the fragrant odor of rosemary will become a most effective household deodorant.

This same method can be used with other natural aromatics such as cinnamon, cloves, vanilla beans, orris root, sandalwood, or peppermint, for example.

A Clean Scented Sweep

Sprinkle the scented water of a **pure** (non-synthetic) floral cologne on the bag of your vacuum cleaner. As you vacuum your carpets the cologne will impart its delightful fragrance to the entire house.

Herb-Sented Candles

Any aromatics of your choice can be blended to make scented wax candles. Sandalwood, for example, makes an excellent addition to a blend as it has a fine aroma and marked fixative properties. It can be used in the form of fine chips, or the oil may be employed.

Or you might like to try frankincense and/or myrrh. Both are gum resins of great antiquity, and were once valued on a par with gold. The Bible states that no less than 20,000 bowls and 30,000 pans for burning frankincense made up part of the fabulous wealth of King Solomon. Today, frankincense is still an important ingredient in fumigating powders, incense and perfumes.

Directions:

1. Melt paraffin wax, add powdered aromatic herbs, or fragrant herb oils, and stir thoroughly. Take ordinary candles and dip quickly in the melted scented wax. Repeat several times until sufficient layers of fragrant wax adhere to the candles.

2. Here is another method: Attach paper clips to the wicks of the candles and fasten to a stretched wire or string, then pour the melted scented wax over the hanging candles. Have a container beneath the candles to catch the drippings.

Lighted scented candles will add a delightful fragrance to the rooms of your home. And here is a tip that will come in handy: keep a candle burning the next time you have company and there is a lot of cigarette smoking going on. You'll be surprised at how effectively it neutralizes much of the cigarette smoke. If the room is large you may have to burn two or three candles.

Clove-Orange Pomander Ball

Stick whole cloves (with the round ball on top) into a small thin-skinned orange until the entire surface is studded. The fruit should be so tightly packed with the cloves that little of the skin can be seen between them. Roll the orange in powdered cinnamon and powdered orris root, patting on as much as you can. Wrap the orange in tissue paper and store it for several weeks in a cool dry place. When the time period has ended, remove the tissue paper and shake off the excess powder. Your pomander is now ready for use. It can be hung by a ribbon or string and kept in a closet to eliminate damp, musty odors, and to give the clothes a delicate fragrance. This pomander will retain its aroma for years.

Kitchen Tips

1. To give your garbage disposal unit a clean, fresh aroma, run the skin of a lemon or grapefruit through the disposal once a week.

2. If you find the odor of cooking fish objectionable, just soak the fish in lemon juice for about half an hour, then cook in the usual way. There will be no fish odor.

3. A few caraway seeds sprinkled in the water in which shrimp is boiling will eliminate the odor.

Paint Deodorizer

To help neutralize the strong smell of fresh paint, place a bowl of chopped raw onions on the floor of each room you are painting. Take a small stick and turn the onions from time to time. (There will be no onion odor either.)

Potpourri for Miscellaneous Odors in the Home

These are botanical substances which are placed in jars to perfume the home with the delicate fragrance of a summer garden. To insure a well-blended and mellow aroma, potpourri mixtures should be kept in a closed container for about three weeks or longer before being placed in potpourri jars. Mixtures improve with age and are comparable to the finest perfumes.

Rose Potpourri.

Mix the following ingredients thoroughly in a large bowl:

> 6 cups dried rose petals
> ½ tsp. orange-mint flakes
> ½ tsp. ground allspice
> ½ tsp. ground cinnamon
> ½ tsp. ground orris root

Pack the preparation in a jar and cover tightly. Allow to stand for at least three weeks, but open the container every few days and stir the contents. Then place in potpourri jars.

To scent your rooms, simply remove the cover of the jar. Once the atmosphere of your home is well scented replace the cover so that the aroma can build up again in the contents. Potpourri mixtures retain their fragrance for years.

English Potpourri.

Prepare a mixture of dry rose petals, lavender flowers, carnations, and any other aromatic flowers. Prepare a second mixture of the following:

> 4 oz. ground orris root
> 2 oz. ground cloves
> 2 oz. ground cinnamon

4 oz. gum benzoin
1 oz. cardamom seeds
1 tsp. oil of rose geranium
3 lbs. of course salt

Place a layer of the dried flowers on the bottom of a wide-mouthed container. Follow with a layer of the second mixture and continue alternating the layers until the jar is filled. Press down firmly, close the container, and let the preparation stand for several weeks. After the time period has elapsed, mix the contents thoroughly and place in potpourri jars.

Note: The possibilities of varying a basic potpourri mixture are unlimited. Spices, dried lemon or orange peels, herb leaves, aromatic gums, herb oils, chips of sandalwood, sassafras, or cedar may be added to any aromatic flowers of your choice. Aside from the dried flower petals, individual ingredients are generally broken up and reduced to the size of a split pea; or some of the substances may be used in the form of a coarse powder.

HOW TO MAKE YOUR OWN HERBAL SACHETS

Sachets are aromatic mixtures in the form of moderately fine herbal powders which are enclosed in small envelopes or tiny cloth bags. They are stored with clothes, linens, stationery, in dresser drawers, chests, wardrobe closets, boxes, and trunks, to keep them sweet-smelling and also to keep them free from destruction by moths.

Along with their fragrance and moth repellant power, certain herbs and herb oils also prevent the fungus growth of mildew and mold that can ruin clothing, linens, and books. These botanicals are invariably included in do-it-yourself sachet recipes, and in some instances they can be used alone.

As with colognes, incense, and other scented mixtures, sachets are generally composed of two main ingredients: the delicate aromatic substances and the "base" or fixative. Fixatives are used because of their strong penetrating odor which strengthens and highlights the more elusive fragrance of the delicate aromatic agents. More than one base or fixative may be used if it blends well and does not overpower the finely scented herbs.

Sachets are best when allowed to stand at least three weeks in a tightly capped jar so that their fragrance may build up and become well blended. The powders are then poured into small envelopes or dainty cloth bags.

The life of a sachet is prolonged when stored in *closed* bureau drawers, closets, etc.

Sachet Recipes

Fragpania Sachet

> 8 oz. powdered orris root
> ½ oz. powdered sandalwood
> ½ oz. powdered khus-khus
> ¼ teaspoon oil of rose geranium
> ¼ teaspoon oil of sandalwood

> Mix powders together, then add the oils and mix again.

Lavender Sachet

> Mix:

> 6 oz. lavender flowers, coarsely powdered
> 1½ oz. gum benzoin, coursely powdered
> ¼ teaspoon lavender oil

Heliotrope Sachet

> Mix:

> 8 oz. powdered orris root
> 4 oz. geranium leaves
> 2 oz. ground tonka beans
> ½ oz. ground vanilla pods
> ¼ oz. heliotrope oil

Clove-Pink Sachet

> Mix:

> 2 oz. powdered orris root
> 1 oz. dried lavender flowers
> ½ oz. deer tongue leaves (vanilla leaf)
> 2 tsp. allspice
> 2 tsp. ground cloves
> 10 drops oil of rose geranium
> 10 drops oil of orange flower
> 10 drops oil of lavender
> 10 drops oil of sandalwood

Spicy Sachet

Mix:

6 oz. powdered orris root

1 oz. each: ground cloves, mace, caraway, cinnamon, tonka beans, nutmeg.

AROMATICS THAT CAN BE USED SINGLY

If you do not want to bother preparing the sachet mixtures, here is a brief list of aromatics that can be used alone to scent clothes and linens, repel moths, eliminate damp musty odors, and resist mold or mildew.

The oils may be applied with a cloth or spray inside bureau drawers and trunks before storing your materials. Or a cloth may be lightly dampened with the oil and hung in a closet or tucked into chests or trunks. Herb oils are strong and penetrating, therefore only a small amount is sufficient for a lasting effect.

KHUS-KHUS

Form Used: Dried Roots—Powder

Khus-khus roots are sold in markets throughout the islands of the West Indies. Natives sprinkle water scented with the roots on awnings and various sunshades, not only for its cooling effect but also for the refreshing and pleasing fragrance it gives to stifling air.

In Jamaica the roots are steeped in coconut oil and used to anoint the body of the bride just before the marriage ceremony.

The fragrance of dried Khus-khus is similar to sandalwood with slight traces of the odor of myrrh. When the roots are kept in closed trunks, dresser drawers, and chests, the aroma is retained for years.

Khus-khus was popularly known as Vetiver in the French colonies of old Louisiana.

LAVENDER

Form used: Dried flowers—oil

This was probably the most popular of all aromatics in Elizabethan times.

Leather book bindings can be protected from mold and mildew by wiping or spraying lavender oil lightly over the bookcase.

PATCHOULY

Form Used: Oil—Powder

Patchouly has a fragrance resembling sandalwood. It can be used in the form of the oil, or the powder can be placed in small envelopes or dainty bags. Clothes and linens take on a highly pleasing aroma—a sort of cedar-like freshness.

The famous Indian cashmere shawls were delicately scented by being stored in wooden boxes oiled with patchouly.

ROSEMARY

Form Used: Sprigs—Oil

This plant was beloved by all from ancient pagan to modern Christian times. It was one of the strewing herbs used on great occasions in Queen Elizabeth's day; the herb released its fragrance as people walked over it. Until recently it was a custom in French hospitals to burn rosemary and juniper berries to deodorize the foul air of sick rooms.

Today it is still a practice in many countries to place sprigs of the herb in wardrobe closets and dresser drawers. It was because of its protective power against moths, mold, mildew, and damp musty odors that rosemary was called "guard-robe."

SANDALWOOD

Form Used: Oil—Raspings—Chips

Sandalwood is a popular ingredient in Oriental-type perfumes and incense, and as a base for sachets and potpourri. The Chinese mix fine chips of sandalwood with rice paste to make perfumed candles. In India sandalwood-scented candles are distributed in exchange for alms during the religious fetes.

Like patchouly, oil of sandalwood has marked fixative properties.

Store the chips or raspings with clothes and linens. Bureau drawers or closets may be oiled in the usual way.

SASSAFRAS

Form Used: Chips

Sassafras retains its pleasant fragrance for a very long time and was a great favorite in the old days. The chips may be used in place of sachets.

TONKA BEAN

Form Used: The bean

Tonka bean possesses a fragrance suggestive of vanilla. In grandmother's day, women carried a tonka bean in their purses, wrapped in a handkerchief, and also kept the beans in dresser drawers and wardrobe closets.

SPICY HOUSEHOLD DISINFECTANT

Many spice oils are powerful germicides, particularly the oils of cinnamon and cloves. Some years ago a scientist named Cavel infected beef-tea with sewage water taken from a collection tank. To one sample he added oil of cinnamon diluted to four parts in 1000; to another, clove oil to two parts in 1000. The germs in each sample were destroyed. But when carbolic acid was used, the strength of the solution had to be increased to five to six parts in 1000 to be equally effective!

A diluted solution of cinnamon oil makes an excellent household disinfectant for bathroom floors, toilet bowls, etc. And it also imparts a highly pleasant fragrance rather than the hospital-like aroma of most commercial sanitizers. It is because of its delightful scent that cinnamon was an important ingredient of the exquisite love-perfumes of former times.

BOTANICAL INSECT REPELLENTS

The effectiveness of botanical insecticides has been attested in a long tradition evolved through the experience of countless people. Many old-fashioned herb gardens had a plot of herbs growing near the kitchen door not only for convenience but for pest control. Tansy, for example, kept ants out of the house. Ticks were seldom found where sage formed a ground cover, or where plots of lavender grew.

The Chinese used smoke from wood fires, punk, and joss sticks to repel insects. The Peruvian ground cherry is employed in India as a useful fly repellent simply by placing the bruised leaves around a room. Thyme, gingko, pennyroyal, and elder are noted for warding off certain insects. The Mexican marigold (*Tagetes minuta*) is used to rid the home of flies and fleas. In Africa, fragrant lemon grass is repellent to the tsetse fly. Cedar, teakwood, and quassia are woods well known for their immunity to insects.

Another traditional insect repellent is the large green ball-like fruit of the Osaga orange tree (*Maclura pomifera*). Yet it was only recently that chemists at the University of Alabama "discovered" that "one green fruit, hedge ball, Osage orange, Osage apple, or whatever you want to call it, placed in a room infested with roaches and waterbugs, will drive the creatures out."

There are over 3000 known species of plants which possess insecticidal properties. In spite of this, the use of botanicals has largely been ignored in modern times, and the more dangerous chemical pesticides have been favored. With current concern over the too-powerful synthetic creations of the test tube, the time is ripe for switching to the more gentle products of nature.

Following is a list of botanicals and the different ways they can be used as insecticides around the modern household:

CAMPHOR

1. A piece of sponge or flannel dipped in spirits of camphor and hung up in a room will dispose of mosquitoes.

2. Powdered camphor or clove dusted into the carpet destroys carpet-beetle larvae.

CEDARWOOD

Oil of cedarwood is effective against moths, flies, and mosquitoes. A box made of soft wood, then painted with cedarwood oil, will repel moths as effectively as a cedarwood chest. The fragrance of cedar closets and cedar chests may be refreshened by spraying them periodically with the oil.

CHAMOMILE

If you cannot enjoy an outing in the country or a picnic in your own backyard without being bitten by mosquitoes or stung by other flying or creeping insects, here is something you can use that will keep you perfectly immune: Make a strong tea of chamomile flowers and let the infusion stand until cold. Then strain off the herb and sponge the solution over the exposed areas of your body, allowing the liquid to dry on. No insects will touch you. (Chamomile has a very pleasant aroma.) .

CITRONELLA

1. Oil of citronella can be sprayed on the garbage can to eliminate flies and other insects. As a moth repellent it is used in the same way as oil of cedarwood.

2. Here is a method of using citronella oil that works like a charm for keeping the picnic table free from ants, flies, mosquitoes and other uninvited guests. Take small cans, like tuna fish cans, and wash and dry them out thoroughly. Pour about a teaspoonful of oil of citronella in the cans and set one of the cans under each leg of the table.

MINT

Mint oils or sprigs of mint leaves will repel flies and fleas. Hang sprigs of mint about doorways, place in the sleeping quarters of the family pet, put them anywhere flies gather.

PYRETHRUM

One of man's oldest and safest insect killers is pyrethrum, a herbaceous perennial chrysanthemum used as an insecticide in China nearly 2000 years ago. In the 19th century it was the secret ingredient of Persian insect powders.

Pyrethrum destroys many forms of biting and sucking insects such as fleas, flies, mosquitoes, gnats, ants, roaches, moths, aphids, leaf-hopper, etc. No insect has yet developed a resistance to this remarkable plant.

Pyrethrum is non-poisonous to man and higher animals. It may be used as a powder, or in a water solution. As a dry powder it can be mixed with flour or used pure and should be puffed around the room, especially in cracks. For use in liquid form, the herb is prepared as a strong decoction and the strained solution employed as a spray.

The use of pyrethrum is not limited to the above forms. It is often burned or mixed with other botanicals.

QUASSIA

The quassia tree is native to South America and the West Indies. It is odorless, but contains a peculiar bitter principle more lasting and intense than that of any other known substance. This bitterness makes it an effective insecticide.

To destroy flies pour a half-pint of boiling water over one-fourth ounce of quassia chips and sweeten with molasses or sugar. When cool, pour the mixture in saucers and place in rooms where flies are most numerous. This herbal solution is perfectly harmless to humans and animals.

SASSAFRAS

1. A strong decoction of sassafras sprinkled or sprayed around the house keeps flies away.

2. Chips of sassafras placed in bowls of fresh fruit will eliminate pesky gnats and fruit flies.

WINTER SAVORY

This is an effective flea repellent. A pad or pillow stuffed with this herb may be placed in the sleeping quarters of the family pet.

MISCELLANEOUS HOUSEHOLD AIDS

Botanical Cleansing Agents

Plastic Tile. To give your plastic bathroom tile a mirror-like sheen, wash the tile with a solution of apple cider vinegar and water, then dry and polish with a bath towel.

Brick Tile. Apple cider vinegar will clean brick tiling around a fireplace. Dip a brush in the vinegar and scrub the tiling quickly, then sponge off the moisture.

Nature's Quicky Bathtub Cleaner. Cut a lemon in two and rub the halves over the surface of the bathtub after it has been emptied. Rinse.

Nature's Bleach. To whiten a wooden bread board, rub it with a sliced lemon dipped in salt. Then rinse the board with clear water and allow to dry.

Lime Marks. (1) A cloth dipped in vinegar, then in coarse salt, acts like magic for scouring away hard lime marks from drinking glasses, fish bowls, etc. Rinse well after scouring. (2) Lime deposits that collect on Pyrex pots or glass coffee servers can be dissolved by boiling vinegar in the receptacles once a week. Wash and rinse.

Chrome Fixtures. Try this for chrome fixtures that become dull with water deposits and leftover cleanser buildup. Soak a cloth in vinegar and tuck it under, over, and all around the faucets, then saturate the cloth again with plenty of vinegar. Let it soak for one hour, then rinse, and the chrome will become bright and shiny as new.

Windows. Old-fashioned cornstarch is one of the greatest and most inexpensive window cleaners. Mix one-fourth cup of corn starch in a half-gallon of warm water. This solution not only cuts dirt faster, but also makes the window glass sparkle.

To Whiten Porcelain. To whiten porcelain or to remove rust from porcelain surfaces, rub with a cloth dampened with cream of tartar.

Copper Pots. Save the halves of a lemon after you have extracted the juice. Dab them in salt and rub on the bottom of your copper-bottomed pots. This will make them clean as a whistle.

Aluminum Pots. (1) To clean the inside of an aluminum pot when it discolors, boil the skin of a lemon or grapefruit in the pot with sufficient water to allow it to boil for at least 30 minutes, or longer if necessary.

(2) Here is another way of removing the discoloration from aluminum utensils. Boil a solution of two tablespoons of either cream of tartar or vinegar per quart of water in the pot for 15 or 20 minutes.

With regard to either recipe, after the boiling period has ended throw the water out, then go over the pot gently but thoroughly with a dampened soap pad. Rinse with hot water, and dry.

Secret Method for Preserving Lacquer Pieces

Try this secret Chiese method for cleaning and preserving the finish on your lovely lacquer pieces: Put two ordinary tea bags in 3/4 cup of boiling water. Cover the teapot tightly, then turn off the burner and allow the tea bags to steep until the water is cold. During the cooling process shake the pot from time to time so that the tea bags will become well soaked.

First remove all the waxes and polishes from your lacquered pieces and dry thoroughly. Then dip a terry cloth into the tea and apply briskly to all your pieces. The real secret lies in the fact that you are not to wipe the tea solution off, for tea contains tannic acid which returns the lacquer to its original gloss.

Orientals who deal in these exquisite finishes claim that lacquer requires no polishes, waxes, or oils, and these should never be used. The simple tea solution is all that is necessary.

Mahogany Stains

Here is a tip that can save you the cost of a refinishing job if your mahogany furniture has been accidently stained by spilled water or alcohol. Rub the stain mark with a shelled pecan nut and the stain will disappear.

Leather Conditioner

The reason leather peels and cracks is that it dries out. If given proper care, leather goods such as briefcases, luggage, handbags, and so forth, will retain a smart appearance almost indefinitely.

Castor oil is a good leather conditioner. Before applying the oil, carefully clean the leather by washing with saddle soap or with non-detergent soap suds. Rub the oil in with a soft cloth or with the finger tips and allow it to remain. It will soon soak in, leaving the leather soft and greaseless. If the leather is in an extremely dry condition, repeat the oiling agair the next day.

Scorch Marks

Raw onion will help remove the scorch marks from cotton fabrics and some other types of cloth material. Rub the scorches with a slice of raw onion and allow to set for a short while. Then soak in cold water. The marks will fade.

Vigor for Your House Plant

When a house plant, especially a fern or rubber plant, is dying pour a tablespoon of castor oil around the roots. This will make the plant green and fresh in a short time.

CHAPTER SUMMARY

1. Aromatic herbs can be used in a variety of ways to add a very special touch of glamor to the modern home.
2. Potpourri mixtures impart a pleasant fragrance to stuffy rooms, especially during the gloomy winter months.
3. Specific plant substances are safe, effective household deodorizers which can replace questionable synthetic sprays.
4. Fragrant herbal sachets are used to scent and protect stored clothes, linens, stationery, etc.
5. Certain spice oils may be applied as household disinfectants.
6. The botanical kingdom provides a number of safe insecticides for use around the modern home.
7. Nature's power-packed herbs can be put to work as household cleansers, stain removers, mold resisters, and as preservers of lacquer pieces and leather.

HERBAL GLOSSARY

Alterative: Indicates a substance which heals a body condition by producing a gradual change toward restoration of health.

Anodyne: An easer or soother of pain.

Antiscorbutic: Counteracts scurvy.

Antiseptic: Destroys or inhibits bacteria.

Antispasmodic: Prevents or allays spasms or cramps.

Aperient: Causes a gentle bowel movement.

Aphrodisiac: Stimulates the sex organs.

Aromatic: Agents which omit a fragrant smell and produce a pungent taste. Used chiefly to make other medicines more palatable.

Astringent: Causes contraction of body tissues.

Bitter Tonic: Bitter-tasting properties which stimulate the flow of saliva and gastric juice. Used to increase the appetite and aid the process of digestion.

Carminative: Expels gas from the stomach.

Demulcent: Soothing, bland. Used to relieve internal inflammations. Provides a protective coating and allays irritation of the membranes.

Diaphoretic: An agent which produces perspiration.

Diuretic: Increases the flow of urine. (Because of their soothing qualities, demulcents are frequently combined with diuretics when irritation is present.)

Emmenagogue: Agents which have the power of exciting the menstrual discharge.

Expectorant: Induces expulsion or loosens phlegm of the mucous membranes of the nasal and bronchial passages.

Febrifuge: Reduces fever.

Homeopathic: According to the principles of healing with homeopathy.

Homeopathy: Briefly stated, the theory and its practice that disease is cured by remedies which produce in a healthy person effects similar to the symptoms of the ailment of the patient— *similia similibus curentur,* "like cures like." For example, peeling or eating a raw onion produces a watery discharge from the eyes and nose, therefore the onion is the Homeopathic remedy for the type of cold characterized by these symptoms. Remedies generally come in very tiny tablets or pellets. Potencies are microscopic. Homeopathic physicians consider the patient as a whole—his emotional and mental states as well as his physical condition.

This system was founded by the famous Dr. Samuel Hahnemann, and has been in use for over 200 years.

Laxative: Causes the bowels to act.

Nervine: An agent which acts on the nervous system to temporarily relax nervous tension or excitement.

Nutrient or Nutritive: Nourishing.

Sedative: Calms the nerves.

Stimulant: Increases or quickens various functional actions of the system.

Stomachic: Substances which give strength and tone to the stomach. Also used to stimulate the appetite.

Tisane: A term used frequently in Europe referring to popular herbal infusions, such as linden or chamomile flowers, etc., which are commonly taken as a beverage or for mildly medicinal effects.

Tonic: Invigorating and strengthening to the body system.

LIST OF HERB DEALERS

The listing of herb dealers below is given solely for the convenience of the reader for purchasing herbs described in this book. These dealers are not connected in any way with the author or publishers of this book. You may write for their catalogs or price lists since they also deal in mail orders.

Golden Gate Herb Research
P.O. Box 77212
San Francisco, Calif. 94107

Harvest Health, Inc.
1944 Eastern Ave., S.E.
Grand Rapids, Mich. 49507

Haussmann's Pharmacy
534-536 W. Girard Ave.
Philadelphia, Pa. 19123

Indiana Botanic Gardens
P.O. Box 5
Hammond, Indiana 46325
(Herbalist Almanac 25¢)

Penn Herb Company
603 North 2nd Street
Philadelphia, Pa. 19123

Kiehl Pharmacy, Inc.
109 Third Avenue
New York, N.Y. 10003

Nature's Herb Company
281 Ellis Street
San Francisco, Calif. 94102
(Catalog 20¢)

New Pacific Products Co.
4064 Marchena Drive
Los Angeles, Calif. 90065

In Canada

Wide World of Herbs, Ltd.
11 St. Catherine Street East
Montreal 129, Quebec
Canada

Index